Everyday Mindfulness for Women

75 Meditations to Help You Find Peace in Daily Life

Courtney Sunday

Helios press

Previously published as *Mindfulness for PMS, Hangovers, and other Real-Word Situations* (ISBN: 978-1-5107-3065-6).

10 9 8 7 6 5 4 3 2 1

Library of Congress Cataloging-in-Publication Data is available on file.

Cover design by Jenny Zemanek
Cover image by iStockphoto

Print ISBN: 978-1-5107-8254-9
Ebook ISBN: 978-1-5107-8590-8

Printed in China

For my mom, who made me believe that writing was a noble act.

For my father, who believed that I could be the CEO of anything (including myself).

For my sister, who reminds me to stay connected to who I was as much as who I am.

For Mike, who owns my heart and encourages my biggest, brightest dreams.

For Theo, who has already proven to be my spiritual teacher.

Contents

Foreword

We live in a time of "I know best." Even though this may seem like a book that is following that thread, I promise you, it is not. Life is filled with enough should, and I have no interest in adding to your pile, or looking at your life from my high horse. I am, however, increasingly interested in mindfulness and how it has helped me move through my life with more grace. (I say this as someone who just fell on her butt yesterday in an attempt to figure skate.)

We do the best we can, and sometimes, we become too busy. We say "yes" when we should say "no." We are exhausted at the end of the day but we can't sleep. We add more to our plates. We ignore our hunger, our voices, our bodies. We plough through. I have done this, and I will continue to do this when I need to learn the same lesson. However, as I have gotten older I have become adept at the habit of subtracting. I don't need one more Facebook friend or party or assignment to prove my worth. Meditation is what has given me this confidence. It is something that sits with me when my partner has been working a lot and I am lonely. It is a companion when I am worried that I am the least successful person of anyone I know. It is a deep relationship through thick and thin as I transform each day. Mindfulness has seen me with stringy hair and weepy eyes, and it has seen me when I can't stop biting my nails or checking my social media channels. When I feel anxiety settling in, trying to get comfortable, I politely show it the door by meditating more.

If I feel exhausted by the shoulds, I figured I must not be the only one. This book of mindfulness is for those of you in the world who don't have time to add one more thing to your to-do list. Mindfulness can be taken on the road, when you are drinking coffee, hanging out with your dog, sitting on a plane, or waiting in line. There are countless moments of waiting in our day-to-day lives. Normally, we use that time to pull out our phones and scroll through pages that we forget immediately after. If I quizzed you on what you saw in those moments, it is likely you wouldn't remember. Those are mindless moments, and although that may be nice occasionally, it doesn't fill us with the same benefits as moments of mindfulness. Think of the emotions you would like to be fuller of: Calm? Hope? Love? Mindfulness is a way of getting closer and closer to the person you know you can be, which may be very different from the person who lost their cool on their commute this morning. I started writing these meditations when I worked for Canadian wellness magazine *tuja wellness*. I found that as I wrote, it became more and more natural for me to be present, which prevented stress from escalating.

My hope is that occasionally you put the phone away to get more connected to your spirit and to your divine self. Moments that arise spontaneously can help you say hello to the part of yourself that fiercely protects your own boundaries—and knows when to take a nap and eat chocolate. I believe that the math equation (nap + chocolate = wisdom) is an elegant theory (and I studied math in University, so you should listen to me).

There is no should, there is no rhyme or reason, there is just you. You may simply want to read this book for entertainment or you may decide to incorporate it into your life. I am not here to preach, I am here to connect with you, as a humbly mindful and constantly curious woman.

I hope that you enjoy this journey of self.

Everyday Moments of Mindfulness for Women

Mindfulness

FOR WHEN YOU DON'T EVEN FIT INTO YOUR FAT PANTS

"I want a perfect body . . . I want a perfect soul," sang Radiohead in their hit song, "Creep," circa 1993. Generations of grungy, angsty teenagers sporting rainbow hair and plaid shirts sang along—I may or may not have been one of them. The grunge era may have passed, but the words still ring pretty true. We want perfect bodies (and this was written before Instagram!). We are always trying to improve, and let's be honest, we often focus on the negative. We wish that our bodies were stronger, smaller, larger, smoother, or sexier. We swear we will do better. We will exercise more and reduce our diet until barely anything constitutes as "clean."

When was the last time you saw your body as perfect?

There has to be an *enough* from time to time. The author William Paul Young wrote, "The opposite of more is enough." We must turn off the media that says our worth is directly proportional to the flatness of our stomachs.

Try to center yourself on the thought that your body is indeed perfect in every moment. It has wisdom and intuition to guide you toward health and balance. Your cells know the right thing to do, just as your mind knows the right thing to do, even if it doesn't always follow it—to eat well and do well, offering you deep acceptance and gratitude for the body you live in today.

This meditation is simple. It's a mantra: "So, hum." I am.

Hear the gentle sound of your inhalation and exhalation. Inhale on so and exhale on hum.

Inhale . . . so.

Exhale . . . hum.

Thoughts will pop up, as they often do. Just come back to your mantra, come back to your breath. This meditation will anchor you in the realization that your body will change, your environment will alter, and yet there is a constant in life. "I am" is the present tense—the part of your body and mind that is grounded and connected.

After five to ten minutes, release the mantra, come back into your body, and gently open your eyes. Enjoy the perfection of your body and if negative thoughts arise during the day, send yourself acceptance and love.

So, hum.

Mindfulness

FOR WHEN YOU ARE PREGNANT (AND FEELING FAT)

It is a pretty remarkable thing to grow a human being. Even so, it doesn't matter how many times someone declares that you are glowing. When you have a cocktail of new hormones and are gaining new chins with every week, you may find yourself looking at your pre-prenatal clothing in your closet thinking, "I will never be able to fit into that again."

There is a great avocado meme that says underneath it, "You're the *good* kind of fat." But this is not often how pregnant women feel, even if their husbands are insisting that it is true. (And husbands who are not insisting—watch your backs.)

It is time to embrace the belly.

Place your hands on your belly, which, depending on the stage of your pregnancy may be quite small or the most obvious thing about you. You are likely already embracing the growing life beneath; that part isn't hard. But as you sit, try to breathe and soften the belly as much as you can. Send love to your belly itself with the warmth of your hands and the attention of your breath. Embrace the body where it is right now, rather than waiting for it to bounce back to what it used to be.

Your changing shape is an expression of your expanding heart. Feel yourself filled to the brim with love, not only for the life inside you, but also for the amazingness that *is* you. Only allow yourself to stand up when you believe this (even just a little).

Now it is time to put on the song that always makes you dance. Then do just that. *Dance.* Dance with your whole body, including your belly. Dance until your cheeks are flushed and you feel uplifted and a little silly. (A little silly is always great for the soul.)

You may need to repeat as needed. Until the next mindful dance-off, go swagger in your sexy skin.

Mindfulness

FOR WHEN YOU ARE FEELING LAZY AF

I was born in 1980. Some consider me a millennial, some consider me Generation X. All I know is that I remember far too well what life used to be like before I was so technologically distracted. What did I do before YouTube and Facebook and iPhones? How did I read books when they weren't conveniently downloaded to my tablet?

I was focused, that's what. Now with all of these technological bells and whistles (the sounds we used to hear prior to ping notifications), it is far too easy for a day to pass where our accomplishments become fewer and fewer, even though we may "learn" small and random facts that we forget soon afterward.

We are all twenty-first century goldfish.

If the day is passing by and you are in danger of having your updated social media feed be your most impressive goal, it is time to take a mindful moment. There is no reason to feel guilty for this "break." Let's be honest, the day thus far was an exercise in "breaking."

Many meditation and mindfulness techniques are built around counting. We learn how to count early, but don't always realize that as adults we depend on the simplicity of this hardwired skill and don't catch ourselves fading away into other thoughts, ideas, plans, and sensations while we're doing it.

Not this time.

This time, I want you to count from ten to one with your breath being the anchor. Every inhale and exhale counts as one of those numbers. When you get distracted (which on lazy days is probably often), kindly bring yourself back to ten. Keep doing this until you feel that your concentration is widening. Maybe you can even get from ten all the way to one, but this isn't a competition; it is mindfulness.

When you are done, open your eyes and make a vow to do something that benefits you more than wasting time on the Internet.

At least for the next five minutes . . .

Mindfulness

TO GET OUT OF YOUR OWN WAY

Saboteur. The name sure is sexy and would make a good title for a television drama. However, in life it's not so sexy to stand in your own way. Even when we know better, sometimes we inexplicably and royally screw up. When you can't figure out why you keep blocking yourself from relationships or procrastinating from moving forward in your career, turn to meditation. Sometimes a whole lot of nothing can get you somewhere.

Sit down and take a few moments to close your eyes, center yourself, and focus on elongating your spine. If you feel uncomfortable sitting on the floor, try elevating your hips by sitting on a cushion.

As you move into quiet, bring to mind an aspect of your personality that tends to get in the way. This may be stubbornness, envy, or distrust. It may not be pretty—don't worry, it's not supposed to be.

As you breathe steadily, allow yourself to retrace this aspect of your personality back to where it started. When we find where the hurt began, we can finally start to heal the scars better.

Once you feel you have sufficiently explored where this aspect of your personality began, sit and try to stop naming, labeling, or judging yourself.

Surround your inner self with love and acceptance.

As you open your eyes, bring your growth forward and be the change you want to see in the world.

Mindfulness
FOR WHEN YOU NEED A HUG

If we all said what we wanted, the world would be a more peaceful place. But many of us don't. We want the people in our lives to intrinsically know what we need. When they don't, we get annoyed by their lack of ability to read our minds.

There is something extremely vulnerable about asking for a hug. I have found myself shyly approaching my longtime partner when I have had a bad day that I didn't want to talk about. Past the age of five, many of us have lost the skill of unabashed hugging. We are deprived of oxytocin (the natural "love hormone" in our brains) because of it, and as far as I know, you can't get oxytocin over the counter.

Hugging is good for the body and mind, just as meditation is. It reduces the stress hormone cortisol. Both hugging and meditation even seem to increase your immunity, which seems counterintuitive. During cold and flu season, apparently, you should hug people *more.*

I'm a hugger. I'll take any study to heart that supports my touchy-feely behavior. If you need a hug from someone, start by asking. Most likely, you will get a yes, even if you are asking a less-than-seasoned hugger. Once you move into the hug, notice the pure feeling of embracing. Pay attention to the points of contact between you and your loved one. Ask the person to stay with you for three deep breaths. Perhaps you can even breathe together, but it isn't necessary.

Just take the time to give and receive, bathing in appreciation for this moment of togetherness.

As a caveat, this meditation might be best to do with someone you know extremely well. You don't want to creep out your co-workers or anything.

Mindfulness

FOR WHEN YOU ARE MISSING OUT

Fear of missing out (FOMO) is one thing, but what if you really *are* missing out?

I felt this acutely when I had to cancel two vacations in a row at the last minute. On the first day, I got extremely good at feeling sorry for myself. I imagined the smell of sunscreen and getting what I like to call "vacation brain," which is when every intelligent, high-functioning aspect of myself takes a hike. I become a little stupid, and I love it.

Without the vacation, I was stuck with this mopey version of myself, who was a drag to be around. I decided to dig into my gratitude practice.

When you are missing out, it is important to notice what you *aren't* missing. Turn on all five senses and turn off your devices. Even if you are bedridden or house ridden or country ridden, you can challenge yourself to see all the good that is around you.

On my unexpected staycation, I made my favorite coffee in the morning and I savored it within the silence. I cuddled with my cat in the afternoon for an indulgent amount of time. I went for a long walk and smiled at everyone who walked by me, refusing to allow any lack of participation to be taken personally.

I realized that joy is a state of mind and it doesn't require a palm tree and Bermuda shorts (although both of those things are nice). The next time you have to miss out on something for whatever reason, try to notice what you aren't missing at all. Whether it is your family, your health, or just the simple sound of a bird crooning outside of your window, it is possible to transform your perspective, enjoy your own company, and focus on the things that are worth your attention and gratitude. In any given moment.

Mindfulness
FOR HAPPY HOUR

There is a trend in the mindfulness world called "mindful drinking." Great craft cocktails and meditation cushions are designed to help people notice how drinking makes them feel.

Well, I know how drinking makes me feel, you may be thinking. *Fan-freaking-tastic.*

As good as drinking can make us feel, many people are concerned with how much they are drinking. The guidelines are not always super clear about what one drink for a woman and two for a man really means. We don't know how often we can partake in drinks after work or happy hour and still be healthy, vibrant people.

Mindful drinking is not designed to make you feel badly about yourself. It is designed to make you stop when you truly feel like stopping, rather than getting another round just for the heck of it or because you have run out of things to say.

The next time you order your favorite drink, make a commitment to not having that drink in your hand the whole time. Take a sip, and listen to people. We get nervous at parties and social get-togethers because we are certain that we have to be the dynamic ones. We will be far more memorable if we truly listen and pause and enjoy the conversation as much as the drink.

Every time you have a sip, notice what the sip is in relation to. Do you just want to taste it, or is it something psychological such as mirroring other people around you or hitting an awkward lull in a conversation? Try to drink when it isn't a mask or an excuse to feel a little less.

When the drink is done, pause for at least ten minutes before ordering the next one. Notice how the alcohol has affected you, and examine your desire for the next drink. Make sure that each drink is savored and that you feel truly present. You may be less likely to have a hangover the next morning, and you will definitely be viewed as a superb listener.

Mindfulness

FOR WHEN YOUR LISTENING SKILLS ARE SERIOUSLY OUT OF PRACTICE

Quick: recall the last conversation you had. What did the person say to you?

A lot of us are seriously out of practice when it comes to listening. We live in a me-me-me time with constant distractions. Listening requires that we step aside from our own ego.

The very act of meditation is listening. Within meditation, we listen to ourselves, the world around us, and even to the space in between sounds. For a world that likes to talk, this opportunity to understand without words can be a welcome retreat. The next time you hear or feel too much noise in your life, try this listening meditation.

Close your eyes (wherever you are, as long as you are not operating heavy machinery). Notice the sounds in your environment without inviting your inner critic. ("That's so annoying! Why won't he be quiet?") Try to notice sounds rather than language: the mild humming of a computer, the gentle tap of a shoe against the ground. Work to notice that sounds are never the same from minute to minute—each sound is unique and rooted in the present.

If you listen hard enough, you will realize that you will not be able to predict the next sound. Any individual sound or combination of sounds is possible. As you listen, imagine you are hearing for the very first time and discard any tendency to predict.

The purpose of this meditation is to draw you into your deeper sense of awareness, reminding you of the richness of the world around you. Listen with your whole body. Listen without thinking. Open your eyes to draw in more of the sensory world while keeping your renewed insight.

Mindfulness

FOR CREATIVE BURNOUT

I work as a writer, which means that I wake up every single morning simply excited to be alive and bursting with creative ideas.

Can you detect the sarcasm?

Creativity is not an endless running stream. Sometimes it comes in huge gushes and sometimes the creative stream is so dried out that I wonder if I would be better suited for some sort of data entry job. During these times, I have faith and meditate.

There is a neuropsychological connection between creativity and meditation. (Don't believe me? Google *The Neuropsychological Connection Between Creativity and Meditation* by Roy Horan). It is a way of refueling without having a creative breakdown.

As you come to meditate, take some deliberate breaths and allow your body to soften. Keep a strong connection with your breath and pick up a pen. Bring it to a piece of paper. Close your eyes and before you do anything, feel the ripple of your breath coming all the way through your body into your hands. Let the pen move as you breathe. It doesn't have to come out with words. Let your breath move the pen. Then with your eyes closed, form letters on the paper. Notice all of the sensations in your hand.

As you open your eyes, allow any and all forms of creative expression to flow out of you. Let it be a free exercise to write, draw, or create without any judgment or expectation. Give yourself time for something to pour onto the page. It may or may not be great, but it is the beginning of reconnecting with your creativity. Be open to being surprised by what emerges. This is a great place to reignite your creative fire.

Mindfulness
FOR DROPPING JUDGMENT

We all try our best to be non-judgmental, particularly if we view ourselves as conscious people. However, this is not always as easy as it sounds. Sometimes someone will hurt someone I love, and the judgmental part of my brain will fire. Judgment! Judgment! *Judgment.*

Point one: don't mess with the people I love.

Point two: It is possible to rewire our brain. Our monkey minds are actually a series of neurons that neuroscientists have called the default mode network, located right in the midline of our brains. When we are all over the place with our judgment, we can be certain that this part of our brains is firing faster than a pinball machine.

It's pretty amazing that meditation can help rewire our brains, even increasing the gray matter and helping us become healthier. We will use this exercise to develop focused attention, a pretty difficult technique. In many cases, we have the anchor of the breath or a word or a visualization—but today I will leave you with your thoughts.

Before you run screaming from the closet of your mind, remember that this is focused attention, an exercise of non-judgment in itself. Notice what you are thinking. Notice the sensations in your body. Notice how you may circle over thoughts or make mental lists or shift positions. You are not trying to fix anything. You are trying to create a little space between what you do and who you are. You are trying to tap into that part of yourself that witnesses things without having to form solutions and fix everything. Your mind is a fine-wired machine that is alive and thriving. You aren't trying to influence it. You are just noticing all of the incredible internal things that happen from moment to moment. Our internal world affects our external world and vice versa.

It is a pretty powerful exercise to start from a place of perception. On some days, meditating like this can help you feel more mentally quiet. On other days, it can feel like the volume has been turned up. In any case, your job is to be attentive rather than judgmental. When you feel that has been reached, even on a small level, welcome yourself back to your life and drop some of the judgment. Allow people to live their own lives and carve their own paths.

Even so: don't mess with me.

Mindfulness
FOR RELEASING BAD HABITS

We all have a habit or two we wish we didn't, from enjoying sleeves of cookies to nail biting. In the past, I have done both of those things. Now, I am perfect!

Just kidding.

Even if no one knows about our secret behaviors, we may find ourselves wishing for more self-control. However, wishing is not an incredibly effective way to make change. Meditating may be the ticket to releasing an unwanted behavior or habit.

A recent study performed by Harvard neuroscientist Brigid Shulte indicated that meditation does indeed reduce stress and changes your brain. Some studies have indicated that meditation can relieve lifestyle problems such as the aforementioned as well as other addictions like smoking or television. I love a good study, especially when it justifies something that I have already found through first-hand experience. Here's what we know: it is possible to reprogram your attitude.

Start your meditation by closing your eyes and counting from ten back to one. If your thoughts are particularly busy and in that time you made a list or planned an upcoming event, start again until you feel you have slowed down.

Once you have calmed your mind, focus on the point between your eyebrows. This point relates to the *Ajna* or third eye chakra, which is associated with perception. Draw to mind the unwanted habit you wish to change. Allow yourself to notice everything this habit makes you feel: from pleasure to shame. Then return your focus to the point between your eyebrows and try to imagine the color *indigo*. This color represents transformation.

As you bathe your mind's eye in this color, imagine yourself being free of this habit. Imagine it were true as of that moment. Notice any bodily changes (tension released or acquired) and emotional changes (relief or apprehension). Keep sitting until you feel liberated and capable of truly transforming.

Go back to counting from ten to one and slowly open your eyes.

As you move forward, keep in mind that every step forward is a step. The journey does not have to be perfect, and you may fall backward before you find yourself truly rid of an unwanted behavior. Use this meditation whenever you need a reminder of what you are striving toward.

Mindfulness

FOR MOVING FAR, FAR AWAY

No matter how many times you have moved, there can be of lot of emotional baggage that accompanies the physical baggage of a big shift. We can get so bogged down by the details that we miss the experience until it hits us in the face. We may find that we miss the way the light used to hit the corner of our old reading nook, or forget where we packed our favorite coffee mug that makes a morning feel bright and full.

If you are feeling nostalgic for the old in the midst of building the new, this meditation is for you. Take a seat in your new abode. If you have no furniture, even better: more chances for you to sit in meditative contemplation.

As you close your eyes, visualize the favorite location of your old place. Try to remember the colors, the light, and any smells. Where would you sit? How would it feel? Imagine yourself sitting in this space. After a few minutes, let the visualization dissolve until you are only left with the feeling of that place.

Carry that feeling in your heart and envision yourself sitting in a new place. It may be entirely made up, or it may involve some of the components of your new abode. Get detailed and specific, carrying over the qualities of the first location into the second. Was it the color yellow that inspired you? Was it the fact that it was a sacred and quiet space? See if the things that mattered can be transferred.

As you take your time exiting the meditation, consider unpacking your sacred self along with your pots and pans. Make room for what is divine to you and your house will become a home in no time at all.

Mindfulness
WHILE BRUSHING YOUR TEETH

Some kids are taught to go through their ABCs while they brush their teeth to make sure they're spending enough time on oral hygiene. You may have even seen those toothbrushes that play a song. (They really should make those for adults.)

With my sister as the firm exception, tooth brushing is often one of the many things we rush through. Let's use our tooth brushing time as an opportunity to bring meditation into our lives. Meditation is merely allowing what is, and paying attention. We can certainly do this while bleary-eyed in the bathroom.

The next time you squeeze toothpaste onto your toothbrush, let that be the beginning of your meditation, as if you had heard the sound of a chime. Start to pay attention to the sensation of the bristles on each tooth. If you normally brush fast, try slowing it down. If you are normally slow, speed it up. Try different directions with your toothbrush. Notice what teeth are easy to get to and which pose more of a challenge.

As with any mindfulness exercise, do not judge yourself as you go. Just try to be in the moment. Every time you find yourself trying to hurry, treat it as you would a thought in a seated meditation: acknowledge it, let it pass, and go back to brushing your teeth. For two minutes or more, try to focus on this activity.

As Zen monk Thich Nhat Hanh says, "Each minute, each second of life is a miracle." Even the monotonous tasks of life can take on new meaning with the perspective provided by meditation.

Mindfulness

FOR WASHING YOUR DAY AWAY IN THE SHOWER

Many of my yoga and meditation students have said "I wish I had time to meditate every day!" If there is no discernible pocket of time, I am not a believer in guilting ourselves into habits. A new habit must be incorporated into the things we do have time for—like showering. Unless you are a new parent, this is a non-negotiable task. All of your co-workers silently thank you for scratching it off of your daily to-do list.

The next time you take a shower, use it as a chance to meditate, to unplug, to do less by just being. As the water runs, take three slow deep breaths to prepare your mind for relaxation. As you step in, bring awareness to your body by noticing the physical sensation you experience as the water hits your skin. Is it pleasant, unpleasant, or neutral?

Notice where you pause. Is it when your back is to the water pressure? Is it when your shoulders feel massaged? This can tell you a lot about which parts of your body have absorbed tension and fatigue.

Imagine that the water can wash away your worries. Slow down your mind. All you feel is the water washing your stress away. Even if the rest of your day is calling, and even if you only have two minutes, try to bring presence to the joy of taking a shower.

What we consider a daily, easy joy is nothing but a great luxury for many people in the world, so be grateful for the fact that you are able to take a shower and be in this place at this time as you dry off. Before you open the door to the rest of your day, take three more deep breaths.

Mindfulness

WHILE PAINTING YOUR NAILS

We use our hands all day long. They are our connection to technology, our loved ones, and our work. They are probably the most overused parts of the human body.

Painting your nails prevents you from using your hands, if only for a moment. You can't read a book or take out your wallet or check your email. For five minutes or more, you have to be in the moment (and looking quite fine while you do it).

The next time you paint your fingers or toes, ensure that there is no music or television on in the background. Dedicate yourself to being in the moment, one brushstroke at a time. Marvel in the color and in the mistakes. For a moment, let everything else fade into the background.

Once you have finished, consider sitting crossed legged with your hands resting on your knees, palms facing up. As you give your nails time to dry, close your eyes and imagine the muscles in your hands relaxing.

Notice if you feel anything in your hands, whether it be dampness, warmth, or tingling. Stay with this sensation for a few minutes, bringing yourself back every time thoughts or noises distract you. When the time is over, your nails will be dry and your mind will be clear.

Best. Manicure. Ever.

Mindfulness

FOR WHEN YOU HAVE TO EAT THE CHOCOLATE CAKE

There are some things in life we want to finish quickly—like any meeting where people say the words "fiscal year" more than once. There are things in life we want to last forever—like falling in love, or enjoying a blissful afternoon with a cup of coffee or tea and dessert.

Desserts are special occasion treats, and at least once a month (or more), there's a special occasion. Whether your dessert is raw vegan or dripping with icing, I have a way to make the moment last.

Meditation can suspend time and help us appreciate activities we already enjoy. The next time you have a hankering for something sweet, take a piece a quarter of the size you normally would. Sit down and take in its appearance—the way the light hits it, the different colors and textures—study your dessert the way a painter would.

Keep the dessert a significant distance from your nose and see if you can detect the aroma. Then, bring your nose a little closer and take a big whiff. Keep inching closer and closer until the smell grows stronger.

Let yourself breathe in the sweet scent, noticing your physical reactions that accompany the anticipation of dessert. Are you salivating? Does your breathing change?

Finally, eat a small piece of the dessert. Let it linger on your tongue for a while, feeling part of it dissolve and coat your tongue. Slowly chew or suck on the dessert, letting yourself notice the way it travels down the back of your throat.

After you take your first bite, sit with the lingering aftertaste. Pay attention as this disappears until you are left with a clean palate. Take a deep breath in and out.

Continue in this fashion, savoring each bite and taking your time in between. Some days will call for a second piece of dessert and a longer brush with mindfulness. However, you may find a smaller piece will suffice when you're spending more time reveling in the sweet side of life.

Mindfulness

FOR GREEN THUMB-LESS GARDENERS

"The glory of gardening: hands in the dirt, head in the sun, heart with nature. To nurture a garden is to feed not just on the body, but the soul."

—Alfred Austin, English poet

Whether you have a backyard garden or some herbs soaking up the sunlight from your kitchen window, you are a gardener. To be a gardener is also to be present. Every day there is change; you can either go with it, or you can get frustrated. If you plan on having many gardens in your lifetime, learning with your plants seems to be the way to go.

The next time you find yourself in the act of gardening, whether you're toiling in the dirt or just giving your plants a good water, take example from what's around you. Things grow and change every day, even when conditions are not optimal. Pests may come and (hopefully) go. There may be more rain than sun, or too much sun and no rain.

There may be weeds that are tougher than your plants.

Sometimes we try to fight nature, and other times we learn from it. Each day you garden, notice what's new with your plant. Notice any changes, however minor, and try to bring gratitude to the theme of change. Move in rhythm with what is around you.

You'll be able to garden like a warrior some days. Other days you may feel defeated. Yet as a whole, things keep growing, one present moment at a time. Focus on what went right today, whether it was an emerging bud or a thickened stalk or new tomato. Every day, every moment, your plants can teach you what it means to be mindful.

Mindfulness

FOR WHEN YOUR TEAM LOSES

If you're not a sports fan, you don't get it. Why the fuss? So a sports team loses . . . doesn't this happen every day?

For the fans who own jerseys and plan their weekends around games, they have declared a team as "theirs." It may be one of the biggest relationships of their lives, and when a person in a relationship suffers, *everyone* in the relationship suffers.

The next time you get the bad news that the score was not in your favor, use meditation to take a step back.

Close your eyes. Cover your ears with your thumbs. We're going to do *brahmari* breath, also known as bumblebee breath due to its sound.

Take a deep breath in.

Exhale for as long as you can, creating a humming sound at the back of your throat without opening your mouth.

Fully concentrate on this sound and repeat for ten rounds or more if you're still replaying the game in your head.

Once you have reduced the noise in your head, remove your hands from your ears and open your eyes.

The game is behind you, and your team will win again—as will you!

Mindfulness

FOR A POLAR VORTEX

Even those inclined to winter sports have to admit: a long and hard winter can be a serious, soul-crushing thing. When icicles are hanging from your eyelashes, you want to curse anyone who has earnestly sung the song "Winter Wonderland." Although the words "polar vortex" feel very modern and apocalyptic, it was Charles Dickens who first coined the term.

Once the winter weather begins to thaw (which I promise will happen) and you are reminded of what honest-to-goodness sunshine looks like, let's get the winter out of your bones. Use this mindfulness exercise to venture out of your hibernation.

Have a seat and sit up tall. Close your eyes. After you settle into quiet, scan your body from head to toe. Really try to focus on each area and notice if any areas feel disconnected or frozen. Try to bring a sense of awareness to your entire body.

Imagine a warm light radiating from inside your heart into every nook and cranny of your body. Feel the warmth hit every bone and every muscle. Feel it course through your bloodstream. Feel this warmth start to thaw any frozen spaces that may have been undernourished in the winter months.

When you feel calm, relaxed, and glowing, open your eyes. Goodbye, polar vortex. It was nice knowing you.

Hello, Spring!

Mindfulness

FOR WHEN YOU AREN'T QUITE WHERE YOU WANT TO BE

I have had my dream job, and still felt uncertain. I have been able to pay my rent, nourish my relationships, and take some time for myself. Yet still something in me was unsettled. I wasn't quite where I wanted to be, but I didn't know which direction to turn.

Have you ever felt this way?

When everything looks great on paper from the outside, it is hard to find reason to complain. These are times when we keep to ourselves when things feel off. We might feel our muscles tighten and think, *what's up with me?* and hold it close to our chests.

This is when it is time to sit. Not to solve, but to calm. Not to decide, but to soften.

Take a seat where your hips are elevated. Place your hands on your thighs at a location that allows your shoulders to fall heavily within your shoulder sockets. Close your eyes and feel your eyes behind your eyelids begin to soften. Tune into all of your senses. Observe the rise and fall of your breath. Get grounded in the body as you drop into the breath. Allow yourself to feel lighter through the crown of your head and through your spine.

Bring your attention back as your attention wanders, especially if that part of you that wants all the answers interjects. This part of you is probably hyper alert at this particular moment in time. They want a solution. Let them know you hear them, but for now, all you need to do is breathe.

"There is nowhere else to be." Repeat that to yourself as you sit. Repeat it until you believe it. After grounding, bring yourself back and give yourself a break, just for once, from moving forward.

Mindfulness

FOR DRINKING COFFEE

You may think that drinking coffee and meditating are about as similar as boot camp and yoga. Think again: there are places where they can cross over.

Meditation is meant to shine light on a deep feeling of inner awareness. It is meant to make you more engaged with the world, not less. Coffee, when used moderately, does the same thing. It helps open your eyes a little more, and if used consciously, can bring you into a more flexible and open mindset.

The next time you have the pleasure of a cup of coffee in your hands, don't chug it back and get on with your day.

Let the taste of the coffee be the object of your meditation.

Deepen your experience of each sip. Note the action of swallowing.

Take enough breaks to notice if you feel a shift in your internal environment. Notice when your body feels the stimulation of the coffee.

If you have thoughts during the coffee drinking, that's perfectly natural, as the nature of our minds is to think. Yet see if you can use the taste of your beloved beverage to stabilize your mind and bring you into a present state.

Every time you get distracted, take a sip and let it wash over your tongue. Let every mindful taste awaken your awareness. You may find you need less to get the same invigorating results.

Mindfulness

FOR WHEN YOU HAVEN'T GOTTEN ANYTHING DONE TODAY

There are days when we have to get something done—a deadline is looming or someone is expecting us to be there. Okay, let's be honest, most days have this particular rhythm.

It doesn't mean we have to like it . . . does it?

Although the sweet parts of life are easy to cling to, meditation teaches us that we must learn to be aware of and accept the not-so-sweet parts of life, like when it is a gorgeous day yet we are stuck at work doing something that can at best be described as mundane.

There is a personal freedom in awareness that may be able to linger during our commute or our early morning wakeup call.

Consider the word *tapas,* which in Sanskrit means "inner fire" or "discipline." This word is often mentioned in the context of meditation in the Vedic scriptures. If you find that you are procrastinating or begrudging your duties, try to find discipline for self-realization.

Make an appointment in your calendar for meditation every day of the week.

Take five minutes or more and just sit. Do it even if you are stressed. Do it when you have a million things to do.

Taking this time to cultivate tapas in meditation can transfer over to other aspects of your life, like those boot camp classes or that paper you have to write for your graduate thesis.

Sit and do nothing . . . to give you the potential to do everything.

Mindfulness

FOR WHEN YOU NEED TO SLAY YOUR JOB INTERVIEW

Today is the day. You have your suit pressed, your notes prepared, and your resume in top form. Yet your palms are sweating and your heart is racing. It feels like the worst kind of first date.

Take a deep breath.

Take another one. You need to find your calm. Especially before you step in to show your interviewer(s) the best version of yourself. This way, even if you don't get hired, at least you can be certain that you did your best as your most authentic self.

To get grounded before you set foot into the building, take a seat or lie down. Start by focusing on your feet. Say to yourself, "I relax my feet. My feet are relaxed."

Take a deep breath.

Move up to your ankles. Say the same sentence with the word "ankles" in place of "feet."

Systematically move your way up the entire body: shins, knees, thighs, buttocks, pelvis, belly, chest, back body, shoulders, arms, hands, neck, head, face. Be slow and selective, taking at least five minutes to relax your entire body. When you are finished, you will most certainly be less in your head and more in your body. Take your confident, capable self out the door to a world of new possibility.

Mindfulness

FOR WHEN YOU ARE FREAKING OUT ABOUT EXAMS

It's crunch time.

Whether you're a full-time student or returning to school part-time, exams are often plagued with stress. I had my first bout of insomnia at University before an exam on partial differential equations. In retrospect, I am so glad I passed that course because I complete partial differential equations all the time. And I totally remember what they are.

Although you can't meditate your way through an A+, you can certainly reduce the stress you experience as you prepare. If you remain in a stressed state, it can interfere with your mind's ability to retrieve information. If anything, you want your brain to be in optimal condition for your exam.

It's important to minimize distraction and focus on what you are doing while studying. Prior to hitting the books, have a comfortable seat (perhaps in the chair that will be supporting you while you wile away the hours).

Close your eyes. Bring your focused attention to your breath, counting one as you inhale and one as you exhale. Then, count to two. Go all the way to ten (it is harder than you think!).

If you get lost along the way, start back at one. If you get up to ten, count backward from ten until you feel that your mind is clear and you are more centered. Studies have shown that mindfulness exercises can improve test scores as meditators have fewer task-unrelated thoughts—sure beats extra time in the library.

Mindfulness

FOR WHEN YOU HAVE OVERINDULGED

Overdid the holiday eating or drinking? As much as our health intentions may sway toward moderate, holiday parties can bring out the human in all of us. After the holidays are over, it can be easy to put our minds on overdrive, devising exercise plans and diets that will get us back to our normal selves.

It is wonderful to plan to be healthy. However, too much planning means not enough time in the present moment. It also often means you aren't being too nice to yourself. Over-planning can be a sign that you aren't accepting yourself as you are—and you are fantastic, even when you have had too many cookies.

Once you've put the fork and champagne glass down, once you've signed up for your spinning class, consider meditation. This meditation is designed to move you away from "overdoing" into simply "doing." We will try the Zazen practice, which is the nature of studying the self by forgetting the self. In forgetting the self (including the self who overdid it) we can learn many things.

First things first. Position your body effectively so that you can be comfortable while paying attention to the body and the breath. Make sure you feel grounded and stable, whether you're sitting in a chair or in lotus position. Gaze a few feet in front of where you sit.

Let yourself focus wholeheartedly on your breath. Breathe in and out through the nose, being with each breath as it comes and goes.

Just be with the breath and then after some time, just *be* the breath. (Deep, huh?)

If thoughts come, let them come and then go again. If bodily sensations arise, let them come and go without clinging to them. According to Zen philosophy, out of the stillness our whole life arises. Your breath will slow down as you continue, as will your reactions to yourself.

Zazen is not about having a goal of any sort; so as soon as you feel you are done, let yourself release the meditation. Let yourself keep your free and clear mind as you continue about your day.

Mindfulness

FOR A SONG STUCK IN YOUR HEAD

It's the era of catchy pop songs. Even if you choose not to listen to the likes of Lady Gaga or Justin Bieber, their music may accost you as you shop, go to the bank, or just live. All of a sudden, you're driving along wondering how "Call Me Maybe" is in your head. And it won't. Get. Out.

Meditation is a way to steady the mind, and what better time to steady yourself than when you are annoyed by your own voice? Even if you're driving, walking, or are unable to sit still and close your eyes, you can do this meditation to get your mind back on track to the more important things in life.

As the chorus of the song repeats in your head, start to repeat a new mantra. *Sat* (prounced sut). *Nam* (pronounced nom). As you inhale, try to subtly hear the sound itself resonating in your breath.

Hear the sound fully: *Sat*. Then draw out through your exhalations, *Naaaaaahm*. *Sat Nam* means "truth is my identity" and it affirms your identity and your highest self. And your highest self probably does not know the Mainstream Top 40.

Look at Sat Nam as retuning your voice. Say it enough times to feel your voice more clearly than any song, then keep the music off for a little while to listen to the world around you.

Mindfulness
FOR HANGOVERS

So you let "just one drink" become "one too many." Now you're paying for it and wondering why alcohol exists. I have a decade of photos with red wine–stained teeth. I may know a little about this feeling.

There are so many techniques out there to rid yourself of a hangover, from "hair of the dog" to greasy breakfasts. Keep hydrated and try this meditation to increase your positivity and awareness so you don't take your mood out on anyone in your path.

Have a seat (or lie down if it's that kind of hangover). Meditation will allow your body to rest deeply, which is precisely what it needs at this moment. If you have partied hard, you also need to rest hard. Take a few deep breaths until you feel a little calmer and a little less grumpy.

Pinpoint a part of your body that is feeling the effects of last night. Start to direct your breath from this place. It's almost like you are breathing from this place rather than from your lungs. Stay there for at least a couple of minutes.

Then move on to another area. Pounding head? Churning stomach? Rather than trying to distract yourself from what your body is experiencing, experience it directly and breathe into it. Take your time, telling each part of your body that you are on the same team. Think of Zen monk Thich Nhat Hanh's simple advice, "Smile, breathe, and go slowly." Particularly on a day when you're feeling slower than normal, these are words to live by.

Mindfulness

FOR WHEN YOU ARE STUCK

There are times in life where you may relish sitting in one place, reveling in your relationship, your job, or just your general place in life. Then you realize that there hasn't been movement in some time.

Uh-oh. Are you stuck?

Stuck-ness is a state of mind that can put any of us into overdrive. What can we do? How can we fix it? Should we take courses? Should we spice things up? Where should we start?

Therein lies the rub. As soon as you realize you are stuck, you are becoming conscious of something within yourself that is dissatisfied. And it is the human condition that we want to immediately turn dissatisfaction into satisfaction.

If only it were that easy.

You may have been living in happy ignorance for quite some time before you realized that things were not as contented as you had thought. If it has hit you like a ton of bricks, this is a sign that all your inner signals have been ignored. Things often appear as whispers before they come as shouts. The problem is that in today's day and age, we don't even have enough quiet to hear our own inner rumblings.

You need to become still. Sit down and feel where you feel stuck. What does stuck mean to you in this moment? Where can it be felt physically? Every time your logical mind interjects with a solution, bring yourself back into your body.

There are times when we are moving and there are times when we are still. Stuck is when we feel that we always have to be moving. Stay and listen. The solution may be more nuanced and quieter than you expect.

Mindfulness

FOR WHEN YOU HAVE MESSED UP BIG TIME

When you watch a toddler make a mistake, they just say the magic words "uh-oh" and then it's all done with. Too bad there isn't such a word in the land of adults. When we mess up, we can spend hours, days, and even weeks reliving the same experience and beating ourselves up.

Let's treat this meditation as the equivalent of an "uh-oh."

The next time you cringe at a mistake, sit and notice where the blame is lying. Is it with yourself? Is it with someone else? Try to just notice without reiterating the story in your head.

Admit how you feel, paying attention to your inner critic. It is okay that you made a mistake. All of us do.

What advice would you give a dear friend who went through the same experience? Meditation gives us permission to be fully human, even when being human is uncomfortable.

Come back to being present, even if your ego is committed to the past.

Come back to the immediacy of your experience. In the now, nothing is going wrong.

Once you leave your meditation, do what you need to do to move forward. Apologize. Work hard. Forgive yourself.

A mistake can be a one-time deal and a way of helping you become stronger.

Mindfulness

FOR BITING YOUR NAILS

"If you correct the mind, the rest of your life will fall into place."
—Lao Tzu

Nail biting, like any habit, can be hard to break (that's an unintentional nail pun if I've ever heard one and I'm just going to go with it). People do it to fight stress but sometimes it's just an unconscious response. Your hands may even go in your mouth every time there is stillness. Or you may be a cuticle biter, unbeknownst to you, until your partner kindly yells, "Stop!"

This is where meditation can help.

Nail biting won't stop if you won't treat the underlying cause or if you don't stop long enough to understand why you fidget in this particular way. It is possible to practice presence every moment of your life, but you can start with when you get the desire to bite your nails (or if you catch yourself with a hand already in your mouth).

At that moment, stop and question how you feel inside. Is there frustration or anxiety? Is your heartbeat slow or fast? How about your breathing? You don't need too much time to scan, but make sure you are being thorough and honest.

Try to feel whatever you are feeling without masking it. If you are feeling nothing but the desire to bite your nails, the addiction is speaking through you. Try to find the real you underneath it. After you have taken the time you need to be and to feel what you need to feel, return to what you are doing.

When you are first breaking this habit, you may need to do this thirty times a day. Eventually it will become less and less until you have healthy nails and a healthier commitment to presence.

Mindfulness

FOR WHEN YOU CAN'T FIND YOUR KEYS

I recently moved into a new apartment. When I was in the process of moving, I grumbled with heavy boxes and shoved things into corners to deal with later until I eventually looked around and thought: *The key to my new place . . . where did I put it?*

Soon I found myself tearing apart my neat work, breathing erratically and acting like a crazy woman looking in the same places again and again. I found myself becoming angry at an inanimate object, then angry at my partner, then angry at myself. It wasn't pretty.

I never found the key.

But I did come back home and think, *Wow, that wasn't cool. I need a key meditation.*

No matter how mindful we may be in our day to day lives, there are unexpected moments that push our stress to the forefront. Keys make our lives easier, but when they are missing, they can throw a whole day out of whack. And therein lay my problem. That forecasting. That assumption that because something slipped up now, it would lead to future misalignments.

I should have stopped looking for the key when I realized that frantically searching in my fight-or-flight state was not working. I needed a calm mind and a spacious mind. I should have sat down and taken two or three minutes to stop freaking out, taken a deep inhale, held it for a while, let it go, and held it again. I should have repeated this, and then allowed the breath to be itself. I should have noticed the pauses between the breath to release my wound-up patterns. I should have stayed long enough to think, *what key?* If I had done that, I may have just found the key. Instead, I medicated with a glass of wine, which has its own abilities to make me feel just fine.

Mindfulness

FOR PEOPLE WHO ARE ALWAYS BUSY

When did we start to prove our worth by how busy we are? When you ask a toddler what he did at preschool, you most certainly won't be hit with a list of amazing accomplishments. It's enough to paint a painting, nap well, and then call it a day.

Until it isn't.

Coming back from a weekend, the first moments at work can sound like a verified competition. The winner is the person who had the least fun and got the most tasks done. If you come in and declare, "Wow, my weekend was great! I did nothing!" you will likely be met with the sound of crickets.

It is time that we stop declaring our busyness as our identity. We are more than what we do and how many Facebook friends we have. Even if we did nothing, we deserve the very best. Start by giving yourself this awareness by reciting a mantra that is built into your very breath. Seeing that we breathe around 23,000 times a day, this certainly gives ample opportunity to find a meditative moment in your day. As you inhale think, *release*. As you exhale, think, *ease*. Then notice that there is a little pause between your inhale and your exhale. In this pause, add the word, *relax*.

Release. Relax. Ease.

Repeat this, even as sensations come up, even as sounds come into your awareness, and even as you insist to yourself that you need to get things done. Leave your dishes in the sink. Leave your email unchecked for a moment. You are busy being a blissful human being.

Mindfulness FOR NON-HIPPIES

There are people who proudly drink kombucha and carry yoga mats with a peace sign on them without the slightest hint of irony. Then there are people who rush by those people—on their cell phones, trying to fit yoga in between the rest of an insanely scheduled life that includes more mudras of the middle finger than of the thumb and second finger.

You do not appreciate being told about your aura or being asked to chant *om*, and the smell of incense does not bring you to a good place. You may be assuming that meditation is not for you, either.

But it is.

Meditation is not just for those who refer to their gurus and rarely wear shoes. Calming your mind is a mainstream idea. It's a way of rewiring the brain. Whether you want to meditate to retain your focus at work or just to feel the positivity you had in your younger days is up to you. Meditation does not have to be a huge time commitment.

In terms of the relaxation response, your brain is not as clever as you may think it is. It's not able to differentiate between an experience and a thought in terms of our blood pressure, our mental state, or even our respiratory rate. When you're feeling overwhelmed by your to-do list, or even dragged down by a recent emotional experience, pause. No need for a special meditation cushion or yoga mat—just sit.

Take a few deep breaths and visualize a place where you've been easily relaxed. This may be a beach you've visited. This may be in bed on a Sunday morning with the paper. This may be fishing at the cottage. Your brain may fight you with this image and storm in with statements like, "I have something better to do!" Bring yourself back again and again.

Visualize yourself in that scene, serenely sitting. And even if you give yourself just two minutes with your mental picture, it's guaranteed that within that time your blood pressure will have lowered and you'll return to your life with more focus and more ability to handle life's curveballs.

Hairy armpits optional.

Mindfulness
WHILE YOU WAIT

There are moments of waiting in all of our everyday lives. We wait for our coffee to brew. We wait for our kids to get ready. We wait for the subway, for our phones to charge, for our computers to start—in fact, when you think about it, it's rare when we're *not* waiting for something.

Even the most patient of us can become a little frustrated with all of this pausing. We may even look at it as wasted time—when we could be looking at waiting as a lot of built-in breaks throughout our day, dedicated to increasing our perception and our attention through meditation.

Vipassana, or insight meditation, is a Buddhist practice that hones awareness of the present moment. The next time you feel the tendency to tap your foot or sigh in exasperation as someone hems and haws over whether they want a soy cappuccino or mocha, notice yourself waiting.

Pay attention first to the things outside of yourself, the people around you, the clock on the wall, the gentle whirring of the coffee maker. Take the time to integrate all of your senses into your waiting. Smell the coffee, listen to chatter, feel the warmth of the room. Then dive back into yourself. If you're still feeling impatient, try to pinpoint where the impatience lies—is it throughout your body, or is it focalized in one part? Pay attention to how your breath is attuned to your waiting and try to control your breathing.

The point of this exercise is to help you remember that you cannot control the waiting, but you can certainly use waiting as a chance to control your reactions to the world around you and decrease your overall stress as a result. Practice enough, and you'll discover a new definition of what it means to wait.

Technological Mindfulness

Mindfulness
FOR WHEN THE WI-FI IS DOWN

The Wi-Fi is down. *The Wi-Fi is down!*

People can quickly spiral into a panic when it comes to their beloved Wi-Fi. I remember when Wi-Fi was fairly new and a disruption in service was almost expected. Now, we are so used to fast speed that we have absolutely no patience when we can't get the information we want, like, yesterday.

Faster speed? Slower patience.

The next time you find yourself with a Wi-Fi "situation" take advantage of the wait to cultivate waning patience. Author and motivational speaker Joyce Meyer encapsulates this meditation perfectly: "Patience is not just the ability to wait. It is how we behave when we are waiting."

Remove your fingers from the electronic devices that they graciously warm all day. Place your hands on your lap. At first, they may twitch. You may fidget. Your mind may say, "But I have to get this *done*!" You will. But now, you will sit.

Notice the physicality of non-doing. If you need to see the point of just sitting, look at it as vacation training. There are people who cannot relax on vacation and it is no surprise. They have no relaxation training in their day-to-day lives.

Now, we're going to work with a mantra. The word *mantra* comes from the Sanskrit word "man" which means "mind." Simply repeat, "slow" as you inhale and "down" as you exhale. You will probably be tempted to peek: is the Wi-Fi back up yet? Give yourself at least ten breaths before returning to your hyperconnected world. If you can do even longer, this will be money in the bank of patience.

Mindfulness

FOR WHEN YOUR UBER IS LATE

This truly is a modern stress and yet one that many people can relate to. Uber is designed to get you efficiently from point A to point B—in theory. Sometimes you watch the car that is meant to be traveling in your direction freeze on the Uber app. You shake your phone. Is the connection lost? Oh, no. Your four-minute estimated time is now *nine minutes*!

These kinds of moments are a way to test your stress levels. If you can jump from zero to one hundred as soon as life brings an unforeseen change, then your sympathetic nervous systems have been the boss for far too long.

Of course, you can always book another Uber, but the same thing may happen. Once you are resigned to waiting, you can use this time as an opportunity for reflection, rather than clocking more hours in dedicated texting time.

First things first. Notice your storytelling. When we are frustrated or annoyed or railing against change, we start to self-narrate. *I can't believe I'm going to be late. What if they start without me? Will I look irresponsible? Why do these things always happen to me?*

Sound familiar?

This predictive voice is not nearly as good at forecasting the future as it thinks it is. Your mind isn't always right, even though it really wants to be. Thank it for its theories. Notice when your mind launches into a story. And return back to being in the moment. How does your body feel standing on the corners of your feet? What does the street that you are on look like? Can you spot the signs of the season that you are inhabiting?

Every time your grumbly voice interjects, take a deep breath to a peaceful, truthful state. You have nine minutes, after all. You will still get to point B—you will just be a little more grounded when you arrive.

Mindfulness
FOR UNPLUGGING

What are you plugged into? For many of us, it's the obvious that first comes to mind: those earbuds or that smartphone or your mother's opinion.

Go deeper and you may realize that there are thousands of things that you are plugged into, whether it be the assumption that you should be married by a certain age or the guilt that you have carried since you moved away from your parents. There are invisible plugs that you probably haven't disconnected in years. What better time than the present to clean house?

Take a seat and close your eyes.

Take a few deep and cleansing breaths to center yourself in the present moment.

As you feel more grounded, bring your awareness to the crown of your head. Imagine circuits coming out of the top of your head, plugging into beliefs, attitudes, and thoughts.

As you get a sense for this, imagine unplugging each one.

Unplug from your company's motto.

Unplug from your spouse's opinion.

Unplug until you are only left with your unthinking self.

Sit in this space for a while, and then consciously decide what you would like to plug back into. Set your circuits intentionally, and get ready for the authentic to come your way.

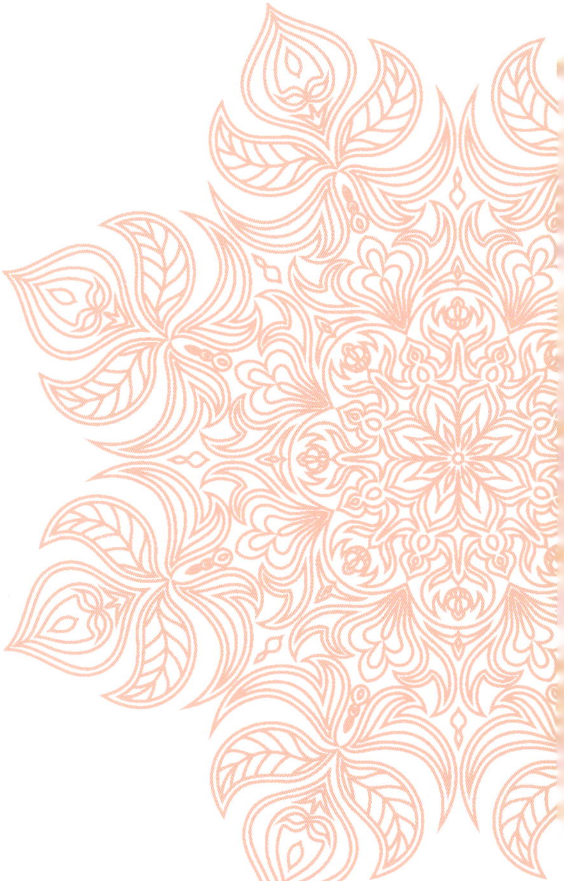

Mindfulness

FOR WHEN SOCIAL MEDIA DISTRACTS YOU FROM WORK

You start the day with the best of intentions. We all do. You may say to yourself, "Okay, first I have to read my email, then I have to get some work done, and then I will check my social media accounts as a *reward*." However, right after your inspiring speech, your rogue fingers click over to Instagram. Those darn fingers have a mind of their own.

Social media is designed to be addictive, and the more we use it, the more it becomes an unconscious act. It can be a powerful thing to limit the amount of push notifications we receive. Some of us may find it easier to refrain from temptation altogether by (gasp) deleting social media apps from our phones.

But this is not a lecture. This is a meditation that knows you live in this dual-plated world. One plate is filled with your highest intentions and the desire to feel connected. On the other plate is your desire to get more followers and likes.

First, let's embrace that you are complex, and that's what makes you awesome. However, a little Instagram break will help you focus and do what you are actually paid to do (unless you are a social media marketing manager, in which case, this is not the meditation for you).

Start by clearing your computer screen. If you have a lot of open windows and tabs, clean them up. Leave it just to the bare basics of what you need to do. Then take one minute to close your eyes. As you close your eyes, be aware of the quality of openness. Notice the way that you feel. Notice the emotions in your body. Notice any sensations. Notice the thoughts in your head. This is not a technique as much as it is a state of being. You are not trying to sweep anything under the rug. You are embracing all of it.

Before your boss catches you, open your eyes. Take a deep breath. Say to yourself, "My intention is to do my work." Try as best you can. If you get distracted by social media, just as when you notice your thoughts in a meditation and do your best not to get attached to them, don't get mad at yourself if you find yourself browsing unconsciously. As soon as you do notice, close the browser, take a deep breath, and start again.

Changing a habit doesn't happen overnight, but that doesn't mean we can't love ourselves, warts and all.

Mindfulness

FOR SOCIAL MEDIA ADDICTS

Are you spending so much time on social media that you think in hashtags? #muststop #cantstop

When you spend more time making social media connections than life connections, it's time for meditation. Put the phone down. Turn it to silent. I swear, it's not going anywhere.

From Twitter to Instagram to Facebook to Snapchat, life moves fast when your fingers are moving at warp speed. Even though we don't have to exercise our fight-or-flight response when we're safely behind a computer screen, our nervous systems don't know any differently. Let's do a meditation to slow things down and get into the parasympathetic part of our selves (all meditation does this). Try the act of vipassana, which is being in the here and now. Whether you decide to practice with your eyes closed or open, work on focusing on everything that's going around you right now. You know, the parts of life that can so easily fade into the background when our phone chirps at us.

Become aware of every thought, of every feeling, and of everything around you at this moment. Notice what you focus on, without judgment. Just let yourself be in the present without a screen getting in the way. This is a good meditation to practice often to honor the art of #disconnecting to #connect.

Mindfulness

FOR WHEN YOUR CELL PHONE DIES

I have been with my partner for many years, but if I were still dating, I would be sure to ask the following question on a first date: "What would you do if your cell phone died and you didn't have access to a charger?"

I think this would give a lot of insight into a person. Of course, I assume the person would lie. That is what many of us do on first dates, in big and small ways. We smooth out our edges and polish the exterior until we are as bright and shiny as can be. We would never be the ones with dramatic reactions or a lack of perspective. Oh no, not us. That is *other* people.

In real life (and not the magical space-time continuum of first dates), when our cell phones die, many of us have reactions akin to action heroes in movies who have just lost their families in a fire. When cell phones first came out, they were cell phones. We had no idea that they would transform into lifelines.

Just for now, you don't have the distraction of pings or push alerts. You have more of an opportunity to feel grounded because of this loss. Tibetan Buddhist Pema Chödrön says "You are the sky. Everything else is just the weather." Close your eyes and visualize a big blue sky. Every thought that comes becomes a friendly white cloud on the surface of your blue-sky mind. You are not trying to overcome the problem and rack your brain for your charger while you close your eyes. You are trying to move away from the grasping, which is what makes us feel divinely unsettled. Sit until you have more sky than clouds.

People pay lots of money on yoga retreats to get disconnected. You just got the same deal for free.

Mindfulness

FOR WHEN YOUR ONLINE SHOPPING IS OUT OF CONTROL

More than once I have declared to myself, "I don't need anything!" and then bought something on Amazon hours later. Hey, I needed those heart-shaped cookie cutters. They were essential.

When there is a massive disconnect between your values and your actions, it means that you haven't spent enough time connecting your mind and body.

Mind, meet body.

Body: "How do you do?" (I imagine my body would be well-mannered.)

If you have had a few episodes with fingers that are faster than the speed of mind, it is time to step away from the computer, or tablet, or phone, or whatever device the kids are using these days. It is time to inhabit your body again in order to feel aligned and connected rather than at the whim of the Pavlovian "click here" button.

Stand up. I am having you do this for a variety of reasons, including the fact that we barely stand properly without a slouch or a hand on the hip or arms crossed in front of the chest. If you feel comfortable and stable enough to close your eyes, do so (you can always stand near a wall for support). Feel the bottoms of your feet. Does one foot have more weight in it? Are you swaying or balanced on one part of your foot??

Then notice your hips. Is one jutting out? Are you leaning to one side or do both sides feel pretty even? This mindfulness exercise is not to try to perfect your form, but to simply practice the art of noticing. (Think of it as an inner "I spy" exercise . . . I spy a right hip!).

Work your way to your shoulders. Notice symmetries and asymmetries. Finally, notice your breathing. Become consumed by the act of being in your skin, and savor each breath. Stand for a couple of minutes. When you are ready to come back, open your eyes and for the love of God, don't immediately go back to your computer. You're better than that.

Mindfulness

FOR WHEN YOUR RELATIONSHIP IS ONLY EXISTING BECAUSE OF NETFLIX

Ruts happen. We would all love our relationships to stay in constant states of ecstasy, but sometimes Netflix and a glass of wine wins. Not "Netflix and chill." Just Netflix.

When ruts happen, aside from the candles and the lingerie and the spice-up-your-sex-life hacks, you can meditate to help rid you of the icky feelings that creep up when you don't feel desired by your partner. Have a seat and take a few deep breaths to settle in and arrive. This meditation will focus on the second chakra, an energetic center that is associated with sex, pleasure, and creativity.

Pay attention to the area around your pubic bone and sex organs. Imagine sensation and energy within your body. Take time to release any shame. Release sadness and guilt, imagining and feeling all sensation in this area. Think of energy rather than anatomy. Go to the deepest layer of being.

Take ten minutes, imagining a ball of orange light the size of a grapefruit around this sacred center. Connect to it. Stories will come and go. Fantasies will come and go. Take back and own your sacred sexuality.

Sometimes our relationships suffer because we don't feel like we have any power. Owning your sexuality and your power will allow you to give yourself what you need, while coming back to your relationship from a clear, blame-free place.

Mindfulness

FOR WHEN CUSTOMER SERVICE IS SLOW

Whenever I hear people complain about slow customer service, I always think they should try working in another country. Throw a language barrier into the mix when you are trying to get your Internet set up, and suddenly you have a lot more patience for the person who is asking, "Can you please repeat your last name?"

The problem with our increasingly fast culture is that even if we had patience once upon a time, likely it has dwindled. We can get ice cream delivered in less than an hour, order books to our door by the end of the day, and watch a new movie in just a click of a button. We have become spoiled toddlers with this convenience. When someone says, "Can you hold on a second?" you may say yes, but there is a part of your nervous system that screams, "No!"

Mindfulness is a way to expand compassion and patience, and can be a great tool to use when you are holding and waiting for help. Rather than letting your voice escalate when you feel your day draining away from you, think *Karuna Hum*. This is Sanskrit for "I am compassion." (And if Sanskrit isn't your jam, just think the English.)

Breathe in . . . breathe out.

I. Am. Compassion.

Karuna Hum.

Putting this statement in the affirmative will help you understand who you are, rather than what you want right now. It will also help you recognize that you are unable to predict the situation of the person who is trying to help you. Maybe he is still in training. Maybe this is her second shift taken to support her growing family. Maybe his mother has just died. This person has offered you a slice of time to move away from "human doing" into "human being." Try to be patient and appreciate the help you are given with gratitude for the available connections around you at any given time, even when it takes a little longer than expected.

Moody & Mindful Moments

Mindfulness

FOR WHEN YOUR HEART IS SHATTERED INTO A MILLION PIECES

If you've had your heart broken, you know it can be as much a physical experience as a mental one. If you haven't had your heart broken, you're a lucky son of a gun. For those currently nourishing their emotionally depleted side, put aside the box of tissues for a moment and have a seat. This meditation is for you.

As you close your eyes, it's quite likely that your mind will be flooded with memories. This will not help in your healing, so for the time being, take a few breaths and let the breaths consume your full attention.

Imagine you are breathing into the space of your heart. Breathe through the front, back, and sides of your heart.

Now take your inhalations as they come and as you exhale say the word "Yum." Really drag out that word: "Yummmmmmm." If it makes you uncomfortable saying it aloud, repeat it to yourself in your head.

The purpose of this meditation is not to fuel your appetite (although if you need a brownie after you meditate, I more than understand). Rather, the word "yum" is associated with the *anahata*, or heart chakra. This will promote healing and set you on the right path.

Plus, it is a fun word to say.

Stay with this sound, letting it reverberate within.

When you feel like you are calmer, open your eyes.

It's time to move forward, one brownie—I mean, meditation—at a time.

Mindfulness

FOR WHEN YOU GOT POURED ON BY THE DAMN RAIN

There was a time when I carried an umbrella with me every day. It was in my purse, and it was my "just in case." It never rained. Then one day, I brought another purse. Guess what happened?

I have lived in some rainy climates and I have lived in sunny climates, but time to time I find myself believing weather reports and not bringing my "just in case." It's one thing to have a light mist on your face. It is quite another to have hair plastered to your face and clothing ironed to your skin. Let's not even talk about the time this happened to me before a job interview. (No, I didn't get that job.)

The thing with being wet and cold is that it can get to you, even after you get dry. It can be very easy to say things like, "Of course this happened to me!" You can use it as an excuse to get a full-time job as a grump. (I know a few of those, although it is not officially on their business cards.) Or you can take it for what it was. Mindfulness can help.

Meditation is about noticing both pleasant and unpleasant experiences. Heavy rain: perhaps not so pleasant. Rather than letting this be a predication for how the rest of your life is going to go, let it be just that—not pleasant. As you allow, you might even notice that there are some amazing things about being in the rain.

Or not. But once you get inside, appreciate the warmth. Bathe yourself in sensation. Experience the pleasantness in the process of getting dry. Notice the thoughts in your head that deviate from the present or revert back to when you were wet and unhappy. It is normal to ping-pong from past experience to present, but when we are not careful, the past can lead our thoughts a lot more than they should.

Pleasant. Unpleasant. Warm. Cold. Everything changes. Let yourself take that rain as a lesson of impermanence. Then try to get back to putting that umbrella in your purse (she says to herself).

Mindfulness

FOR WHEN YOUR PAIN WON'T GO AWAY

If you have been dealing with pain for longer than twenty-four hours, chances are that your patience is wearing thin. We may have patience for other people in our lives, but patience with ourselves and our bodies can be a lot more complicated.

If, internally, you are giving your pain the middle finger, it is time to meditate. This meditation was inspired by a time I went to an acupuncturist in quite a bit of pain. On my way out, I was chatting with the receptionist about how frustrated being incapacitated made me feel. My acupuncturist came from behind a curtain and said, "I heard that. Give your body time."

What was she, some sort of wizard?

Maybe it was the fact that I had just trusted this woman to put needles in me, but I found myself heeding her advice. I listened to the voice inside me that wanted to evict my pain without understanding its cause or its lesson. It doesn't mean that my pain dissipated. But my fight with it started to.

If you are finding it hard to be comfortable, start by finding a position that is perhaps less painful than others. As you find this shape (and it may be quite unique, depending on your condition), close your eyes and find three sounds around you. Right afterward, find three neutral body sensations. Then ask for three images to appear.

Now do the same thing two times. Two sounds, two body sensations, two images.

Then one sound, one sensation, one image.

Go back to three. Then two again. Then one.

Repeat this process for as much time as you have, or until you feel some of the gripping that comes from the fear of forever-pain dissipate. I am not looking for you to stand up from this meditation crying out, "I am healed!" (But if you do, I accept bank checks and credit cards.) I am hoping, however, that it will help to carve a new neural pathway and thus give less power to the pain receptors of your body.

Here's to you and your healing.

Mindfulness

FOR WHEN THE FUTURE LOOKS BLEAK

You may have been doing perfectly fine for some time, until a shocking change turned everything into "before" and "after." It may have been a death, a political upset, or the loss of a job. It could be so many things.

All you know is that you no longer know that optimistic person who once thought everything was going to turn out as expected.

You can listen to Bob Marley's "Three Little Birds" on repeat, but it is time to convince yourself that you have never been able to predict the future, and you haven't gained that ability overnight. I know it's hard. I have been guilty of moaning, "This is never going to *end*" to my partner, who feigns patience and brings me a cup of tea. (Tea helps.)

It's times like this that make meditation necessary. Meditation needs to be done regularly, just like a workout. You don't go to the gym once a week and think, "That should do it." If you have an interest in gaining perceivable muscles, you go regularly. Your brain, the muscle, is exercised a lot, but have you given it any rest days? Muscles repair during rest, and all of the clouded perceptions about your future may be a result of an overactive mind.

Sit down. Lie down. Just get down. This one is simple. Find the breath within your body. Breathing in, think "present moment." Breathing out, think "only moment." The first few rounds you might fight with yourself. Your mind may scoff at the simplicity of this statement and draw you back into forecasting. Simply return back.

"Present moment."

"Only moment."

"Present moment."

"Only moment."

Set a timer for as much time as you have. Hopefully, once your eyes open, your brow will be less furrowed and you will be less likely to let everyone around you know that the end is nigh. (PS: People generally don't appreciate that. Do this meditation for them.)

Mindfulness

FOR BACK PAIN

There are many causes of back pain, but chronic stress is a critical one. When it can be hard to let go in life, our back muscles can physically respond to this by gripping and tightening.

I say this as someone who does lots of yoga and movement, and yet is occasionally sidelined with debilitating pain. I sometimes take this pain as an opportunity to reconnect with myself; to slow down and soften with a meditation practice that honors my present state. (I also take it as a chance to rail against the unfairness of the whole situation, but let's focus on the grounded version of me, okay?)

Make yourself very comfortable and then close your eyes. You may not be feeling terrific in your back. That's okay. Meditation is not designed to "distract" you.

Scan your body from the top of your head downward toward your feet. Take it all in, taking the time to connect with your body in whatever state it is in.

As much as you can, let yourself relax.

Feel your breath, without forcing your breath. Let it happen naturally.

Feel your heart beat.

Feel how alive your body is, right now, even with this pain.

Connect with the intelligence of the body. It knows what to do without you telling it. It is kind enough to give you a message. It is asking you to realign and reconsider. It is asking you to listen.

Your body knows how to heal.

As you relax everything in your body, let the natural healing process of your body take over. Feel the area of your back that hurts and try to imagine making space there. Notice if there is any gripping or emotions surrounding this area. Try to let it go as much as you can, and be kind to the pain that remains.

Later on, you can of course do all of your treatments: your acupuncture, your Epsom salt baths, your massage. Yet for this meditation, just give your back love and attention for as long as you possibly can.

Mindfulness

FOR WHEN YOU ARE IN A BAD MOOD

Some people believe that if they could just get rid of their difficulties, they could really meditate. However, difficulties actually enhance our experience of meditation. In bringing full awareness to our emotions, we can then be open to the lessons we need to learn.

Yes, this means you. This means all of us.

A belief for many meditation practitioners that may help you feel better about this process is that consciousness has been and always will be there; it just has to be recognized. Before we try to let go, we must recognize where we are in the moment. This is easier to do than trying to chant "om shanti shanti" while being filled with annoyance or frustration.

On your terrible, horrible, no good, very bad day, take a seat. What we're trying to slow down in our mind is the tattletale voice. The voice that says I'm mad because so-and-so did this. In this moment, deal with your emotions without inviting anyone else in.

When you feel something, label it. If it's anger, feel your anger and acknowledge your anger without fueling it. Try to silently chant "anger, anger, anger," and then notice the parts of your body that respond to this word and emotion. It could be held in a clenched jaw or closed fist. Bring awareness to this area.

What is the energy of anger like? How does it change your breath? Examine it fully.

Try to release the if-only mind. The part of you that thinks, *if only I weren't so ____, I would be able to meditate*. If it comes up, chant "if only, if only, if only" rather than following the thought to completion.

See what rises on your worst of days; feel it in your body. Eventually, it will pass. Our emotions and bad days are (luckily) impermanent, as is everything else. This day, too, shall pass.

Mindfulness
FOR JEALOUSY

The green-eyed monster. It can rear its ugly head in all of us, even the people who claim that they "never get jealous" while smugly eating their salads.

Why can the person next to us in yoga class touch their face to their shins when after years of practice you can barely get to your feet? Why can your friend eat everything and still fit into sample sizes? Why did your coworker get the promotion when he is less experienced than you?

Scientists have found that the part of the brain that detects jealousy is the exact part of the brain that detects physical pain. This gives insight on why it doesn't feel great to be envious. Who we are in little moments can ultimately add up to who we become. Let's knock this envy out of the park with meditation.

When you find yourself obsessing about what someone has and what you do not, take a comfortable position. Then take a deep breath and let that deep breath fill you up completely. Hold your breath for a few seconds, and then let it go. Repeat a couple more times and repeat these phrases:

> I feel compassion and love for all beings.
> I feel compassion for those who are less happy than me.
> I am loving toward those who are happier than me.

You can certainly make these phrases your own with the area you are struggling with. Saying it the first few times might involve some resistance. The more you practice, the more it will become your truth. We all have the capability to change from the inside, and that is truly where peace begins.

What green-eyed monster?

Mindfulness

FOR WHEN YOU ARE OBSESSING OVER YOUR EX

Sometimes the reason we can't get over a breakup is that we keep going over conversations in our heads. We constantly review what we said or he said or she said (or all of the above), made even worse by the ability to see how happy they look on their social media accounts. (*Who is that person in their picture?*) I thank my lucky stars I am old enough to remember a life without social media.

We may cut ourselves off, then find our fingers drawn to the keyboard, drawing our minds back into drama. If your mind is sounding like a broken record because of an obsessive thought process, it's time to bring your meditation skills to the table.

Take a patient attitude. If you are forceful and judgmental with yourself, you will feel stuck in the repetitive thought process (and even more stressed out).

As you inhale, invite yourself to be open to a bigger experience than your obsession.

As you exhale, imagine clearing away some space in your mind.

Begin to make your inhalations on a count of four and exhalations on a count of eight. If this feels beyond your capacity, try inhaling for a count of two and exhaling for four until you become relaxed enough to increase the count.

After a few minutes, bring in a breath retention. Inhale for four. Retain the breath for seven. Exhale for eight. This type of breathing is not only a natural tranquilizer for the nervous system but also a way to restrain reactivity.

It may only take a few breaths before you find yourself moving away from your recycled thoughts. If you need more time, take more breaths. Become the owner of a more spacious mind.

Mindfulness

FOR WHEN YOU HAVE PMS

This one is for all the ladies in the house . . . or the sensitive men. (Side note to sensitive men with their PMSing ladies: do not mistakenly leave the book open to this page, unless you want all hell to break loose.)

In gym class, I remember learning about menstruation with fascination and horror. I hadn't yet hit puberty, so it wasn't my concern.

Until it was.

PMS hits some women harder than others, but all of us have had an experience where we have watched a kitten on YouTube, crying hysterically. (No? Just me?) Meditation teacher Paula Tursi says, "What feels like an unsuccessful meditation is actually highly productive when you're allowing whatever is, to be. How we deal with frustrating moments is how we deal with life." And what is more frustrating than feeling like your hormones have taken you hostage?

For this meditation, set a timer for at least ten minutes. Make yourself super comfortable. As you close your eyes, take a moment to relax in the space behind your eyes. Don't rush yourself as you take a slow shift out of your head and into your body.

As you sit there, check in on your body first, breathing into anything that feels particularly wound up. Feel what your emotions are, giving yourself plenty of time to unravel your honesty. Feel where your emotions may be stuck. Whatever is there, be with it. Are you crampy? Are you ticked off? Be those things. Exhale into those things. Make space for it and you will find the stuck energy dissipating. Feeling. Being. Full breaths in and full breaths out. Open your eyes, grab a hot water bottle, and embrace those adorable kitten videos.

Mindfulness
FOR INNER STRUGGLE

Ever feel or experience something that makes you think, "This needs to go away immediately?" Whether you're forcing inner peace, a smile, or fighting back tears, how well is that working for you? Let's accept where we are and what is going on together.

Interestingly enough, the more that we allow what is occurring, the more it will be given an opportunity to fade. You know the phrase, "What we resist, persists." Well, it means that the more we try and force the exit of a mood, the more it will attempt to highlight its presence. Even if you're mentally able to get rid of the emotion you're trying to hide, your body may cling to it until it presents itself physically as anything from back pain to chronic headaches.

Take a seat.

With eyes closed or downcast, notice where you are. Recognize whatever arises, accepting its appearance or disappearance. Let go of believing you should be somewhere else emotionally, mentally, or physically. Be open to every attribute of your experience as you sit.

Don't censor anything. *Allow everything.* The pleasant and the unpleasant. The neutral. You can observe it all equally. This inner attitude is nonjudgmental. It may take a while to cultivate, but when you feel that you have opened up your mind to the best of your ability, sit in that space. Become a curious being who can let each moment be. This doesn't mean that you can't take steps once you open your eyes to a different path, a different emotion, or a different mindset. But for now, as you sit, let it be simple. Just let it be and maybe you will realize that what you feel is not forever. It has its time.

Mindfulness

FOR WHEN YOU JUST DON'T KNOW ANYMORE

There are rare times in life when we know exactly how to move forward or who to be with or who to be. Times when we don't question our place in life and where we are going.

Notice I said the word rare when I spoke of these times. Even so, we cling to the idea of knowing. When it goes, we mourn its presence. We wish to have all the answers, especially when they are to our own questions.

When there is something that is nagging at you, begging to bc known or figured out, this is a good time to meditate. Meditation reminds us that we don't always have to hurry the process. We can wait patiently and listen for the answers to arrive in their own time.

For this meditation, have a seat and make yourself comfortable. Relax your pelvis into the earth. Take a big, deep, full breath and feel it in your bones. Listen to the sound of your breathing.

We will do the beginning of a meditation called Isha Kriya. When you inhale, think, *I am not my body*. When you exhale, think, *I am not even my mind*. Repeat the Isha Kriya quietly to yourself for five minutes. If you have time, repeat these phrases for even longer. Repeat until you realize that there is a part of you that is all knowing, a part that you can access beyond the overly analytical, thinking self.

Come into silence, releasing the mantra as you release your expectations.

Mindfulness

FOR WHEN YOU ARE BEING HARD ON YOURSELF

Author Eckhart Tolle has an infectious laugh. He may deal in the realm of mindfulness, but he finds a lot of things in life funny. One thing he finds funny is that most meditators put in so much effort to control the experience and manufacture a specific state.

Sometimes we think more than others. Sometimes we worry more than others. If we try to ignore how we are really feeling, the feeling wins and it becomes bigger. If we sit with ourselves and try our best to let thoughts come and go, we are meditating and we are also allowing ourselves to be, which is the opposite of effort.

The most common thing I hear from my meditation students is that they are "not good at it." Guess what? No one is, without practice. No matter what the situation, the next time you find yourself being hard on yourself, have a seat. Close your eyes and take a moment to observe your experience. Hear the sounds around you. Notice the thoughts coming through your head, and try to imagine that there is a space beyond the thoughts that is silent and accessible. Try your best to access this space.

If you find yourself getting agitated or frustrated during meditation, remember that some days will be easy and some days will be harder. Let yourself try the art of non-effort. If the thinking mind is really strong, let yourself think. Even if you have a few seconds of pure presence, this is a success. This is why we are really here.

Don't take it all too seriously. Find the part of yourself that doesn't need to be the best. Release some of the weight of your achievements from your shoulders. As you feel lighter, slowly blink your eyes open to return to the world.

Mindfulness

FOR WHEN THINGS ARE GOING WELL FOR YOU

We have all heard that misery loves company. Joy, however, can also sometimes feel isolating. Do you become one of "those people" who splashes it over social media until even your friends are sick of you? Or do you keep it to yourself, choosing to save only your complaints for public consumption?

We are consistently told not to bottle up our feelings, but guess what? Joy is a feeling. It is not shameful. Meditation is the art of exploring what is, and this includes the splendidly happy times.

The next time you find things are going swimmingly, don't gloss over it. Don't tell yourself "this won't last." Don't forecast what your joy will turn into. Joy doesn't have to be shared to be real. It can be relished and explored, unabashedly.

Take a seat to examine what your joy feels like. Is it an energetic joy, or a mellow contentment? Is it concentrated more in one area of your inner body, or is it spread throughout? Get curious. As with any meditation, if you get distracted, come back to this settled and contented feeling. You may feel your joy increase as you sit, or it may decrease, or it may stay exactly the same. Watch it transmute and evolve within you.

After a few moments, think to yourself *Ananda (Ah-nuhn-da) Hum*. This means, "I am bliss." Repeat it over and over as you sit in silence. Meditation helps us understand that joy doesn't have to be connected to an external circumstance. We can just simply *be* joyful.

Take that feeling of joy with you. The world needs it.

Mindfulness

FOR WHEN YOU ARE SICK (AND FEELING SUCKY)

When we feel healthy, it's easier to unroll our yoga mat or go for a run, appreciating the strength of the body. But what about those times when, even though the sun is shining, your body is not cooperating with your ultimate plan of wellness? Allergies can kick in, a nasty cold can take effect, and all of a sudden, your mindfulness can be boiled down to the mantra, "screw this." Sometimes negativity can be as pervasive as the side effects of sniffling and drowsiness. This we can do something about.

A very important part of the healing process is to get comfortable, so begin this meditation by putting your feet up.

It may be difficult to breathe, so don't focus on your breathing. In fact, don't try to resist being sick at all, bemoaning what it felt like to be healthy. This in itself can make the virus thicken to make itself heard.

Hear your virus. Envision where you feel it the most. Don't be angry with it; try to be at peace with it. This is hard for us movers and shakers. At peace does not mean you are giving up on your health for good. It is just realizing that this rest is a part of your health as a whole.

After envisioning where your virus is, see if you can feel a part of your body that is unaffected. It could be your toe. Focus on that point, and imagine the healing potential of your body expanding.

Imagine the same feeling you have in that unaffected part reaching to the rest of your body. And then rest.

Rest without distraction. Heal without the television. Give yourself time.

Mindfulness

FOR WHEN THE WORLD IS AGAINST YOU

Most of us have a friend who seems more surprised when things go right than when they go wrong. "This always happens to me" might be their common glum refrain. However, they might want to consider the law of attraction—so much of who we are and how we feel is reflected right back at us. So the next time you are certain that the cards are not in your favor, have a seat.

In the midst of a busy and rushed existence, it can be hard to detect the beauty and joy that is always present around you. Rather than being stuck in your own head, try looking outside yourself to come to a present moment of awareness.

Think silently to yourself the word *om*. Every time you find you are distracted by your thoughts or by noises in your environment, come back to *om*. You probably have heard this sound, even if you have never set foot in a yoga studio. This mantra is a sacred sound that honors the notion of connectedness to the whole universe. It's even thought to be the sound of the universe.

After five to ten minutes, release the mantra and open your eyes. As you go about your day, notice your connection with the energy of the world around you. This will reverberate into your core, giving you the opportunity to let go and bring forth better days ahead.

Mindfulness

FOR WHEN YOU CAN'T MAKE SENSE OF THE WORLD

It can be easy to feel disillusioned when the world is in inner turmoil. How can you sit in meditative bliss when there is war and famine and even challenges within your own family? Isn't that selfish?

The Dalai Lama and other spiritual leaders believe that hope is the antidote to despair. Hope is different from blind optimism or even reluctant pessimism. Hope is the chance to see the world as it is, warts and all, and achieve a wider perspective. It is a way to harness faith that there is no hopeless situation.

Mistaking the inner world for the outer and the outer world for the inner is one thing that mindfulness training tries to unmask. Meditation and mindfulness might seem like selfish, solitary activities from the outside, but in truth, they are designed to help us feel more connected. It's next to impossible not to be affected by reading something about someone else in the news. The next time you are feeling awash with emotion because of the affairs of the world, take a step back and have a seat. As you deepen your breath, feel yourself take in some of the weights that people around the world are carrying. Accept your own empathy.

As you exhale, imagine sending hope.

Inhale, take in some of the world's weariness.

Exhale, give out your greatest faith and confidence.

We are not working here to control life or to fix anything. We are working to become better people who can afford to give more of ourselves to the world.

Mindfulness

FOR WHEN YOU ARE CRABBY

I'm going to tell you a secret. I have been crabby lately. I tell you this in the strictest of confidence, because when I am crabby, the last thing I want to do is admit said crabbiness. I would rather wrinkle my nose and suck all the joy out of my voice and pretend that "I'm fine."

Everyone knows I'm not fine, but I will be damned if I admit it out loud.

At moments like this, my partner likes to remind me, "Hey, you're a meditation teacher. You teach people how to relax." To which I either a) roll my eyes, or b) smile sweetly and say "I'm also human."

I'll tell you another secret: he is right. (Hopefully he will never read this.)

It is one thing to use my mindfulness practice in the best of times, and quite another to use it in the worst of times. What I really should do in moments of crabbiness is go into a room, close the door, and practice the breath of joy.

The breath of joy is a yoga technique that not only makes you feel more energized, it also has the potential to exorcise the grump. First, you breathe in one-third of the way, lifting your arms in front of your body to shoulder level. Second, you breathe in two-thirds of the way, swinging your arms to the side at shoulder level (like airplane wings). Third, you breathe in the rest of the way, swinging your arms over your head.

Then comes the fun part.

Exhale fully, shouting, "Ha!" and bending the knees as if you were doing a squat and throwing your arms behind you. Repeat all of these things five times, ten times, or enough times until you feel like you are throwing your attitude behind you. When you are done, your cheeks should be flushed and you should have some semblance of a smile.

Get back to your day. Take two.

Mindfulness

FOR WHEN YOU HAVE RESTING BITCH FACE

Elf has become my favorite Christmas movie. It makes me cry every single time and it feels like pure holiday joy. One of the lines that Will Ferrell says always gets me. "I just like to smile . . . smiling's my favorite."

What an awesome thing to say.

Some days, it feels like the whole world is smiling with you. In others, it feels like the world is scowling at you and you'd do anything for a genuine "How are you doing today?" kind of smile. You may have even caught your own face in a mirror and thought, "Damn, that person looks mean."

Resting bitch face. It's a thing.

One of the most famous Tao meditation practices is known as the "inner smile." Ever smiled at your liver? Give it a shot on a day when you feel that you and the world are not on the best terms.

Sit comfortably and tall, allowing the muscles of your neck and face to relax. Come into the present moment by taking a couple of deep, steady, and controlled breaths. Start to let the corners of your mouth lightly lift. This should be a subdued Mona Lisa smile that supports the relaxation of your face.

Bring your attention to the center of your brain or the point equidistant between the ears. In Taoism this is known as the Crystal

Palace, the place between the pineal and pituitary glands. Feel the energy gathering in this place.

Direct the energy from the Crystal Palace to your eyes, imagining your eyes becoming affected by the smile on your lips. Let your eyes shine, just like when you're around someone you love. Direct that love and that smile inward.

Continue to smile throughout your body, perhaps directing it toward an area that needs healing or an area that you rarely give attention to (this is where your liver comes in). Continue to direct smile energy throughout your body until the slight smile on your face feels natural.

Then go spread that sweet look around town.

Mindfulness

FOR WHEN YOU ARE WORRYING

When someone in my life is sick or unhappy, much of my mindfulness training goes out the window. I worry. I wonder how I can "fix" it. I Google—man, do I Google. This probably accomplishes less than nothing. After all, no one gets better and says, "It was your worrying that got me through the dark days."

A day of worrying is exhausting. It is more exhausting than a strong workout or a red eye flight or a screaming baby (although worry and screaming baby are often birds of a feather). If you have found yourself in the spiral of worry, it is time to become present. I am not asking you to be mindful in an attempt to obliterate the reality of your situation. Rather, I am hoping that you recognize that a worry is a thought that can embed itself into your body.

Worry is actually a pretty good way to verify that just because we think something doesn't mean that it is true. We know this in other situations, but worry is fierce and has the power can convince us that it is the only logical way of thinking.

Step aside, worry. Step aside.

This meditation is best done with as few distractions as possible. Take a moment to sit down and get comfortable. (When I need some TLC, I sit cross-legged on the couch with a blanket wrapped around me.) Close your eyes and begin to relax parts of your body, especially the tight spots like the lower back, shoulders, and jaw, or parts that are noticeably tense or in the process of healing. Try not to resist your moment of relaxation; this can give worrying more energy.

Make a connection with your breath and let your breath break those chains of worry and powerfully bring you back to present. Your mind-made worry blocks you from the truth, but as you become present, worry has less and less room to grow. Honor the unique path you are on and feel your feelings without judgment. This version of you is what the person in your life needs, which will be far more healing than ample time with a worrywart.

Mindfulness

FOR WHEN THINGS AREN'T GOING YOUR WAY

If you are having one of those days where the world just doesn't seem to be on your side, it is time to flip the equation. You are more powerful than you realize, and although meditation won't make you into a magician, it will give you some perspective.

Take a moment out of the madness and find some open space in a quiet room on a yoga mat or even in a bathroom stall if need be. Bring your phone with you (this isn't how you imagined your meditation would go, is it?).

Find an app on your phone that has a metronome. There are tons of free ones, and if you are flummoxed, you can listen to a constant beat on YouTube (oh, YouTube, what did we ever do without you?).

As you close your eyes, settle into that constant rhythm, counting second by second, marking each unit of time with precision. Begin to match your inhalations and your exhalations to the beat. Make sure it is a count that you can sustain, yet long enough to require your focus. If you normally breathe in for a count of five, make it six, for example. Six breaths in, six breaths out. Six breaths in, six breaths out. Continue to breathe in this way until you feel that your breath is the same.

Let all of your thoughts melt away for a moment. Whether things are going well or going poorly, you have this moment. Whether you have taken ten breaths or one hundred in this way, this technique has the ability to ground you and give you a fresh start. Get off that mat or out of that stall and back into the world to start again. Consider it to be a little bit of magic.

Mindfulness

FOR WHEN YOUR NERVES ARE SHOT

By the time we become adults, we know many things. At the very least, we know how to tie our shoes and make toast. There was a time in your life when these accomplishments would have been nothing short of miraculous.

Hopefully by now you also know a little something about yourself. What makes you tick and what makes you ticked off. The more you know yourself, the more you can predict when you need a little space for the safety of everyone around you.

This meditation is for the days when you don't want to be mean, but if someone as much as looks in your direction, God help you, you *will* be mean. It is for the days when you are generally annoyed, rather than annoyed at someone in particular. It is for the days when you haven't realized that your jaw has been clenched until you look in the mirror and wonder why your grandmother is looking back at you.

For the good of the world around you, take a seat. Or lie down. Be comfortable, and before you close your eyes, get connected to the Internet to find the sound of a gong; make sure the sound plays for at least five minutes. Then close your eyes and become bathed in the vibrations. Notice the silence that enters the soundscape after the gong dissipates. Notice if you are trying to anticipate when the next clang will hit your eardrums. For now, just listen and enjoy.

After the gong stops, sit in silence for a moment and hear the silence. There may be other sounds that run into the silence (when I did this meditation, my cats meowed and my partner yelled, "Babe, do you know where my towel is?"). No matter. Just listen and allow yourself to be still. This mini mindful break will allow you to come back into the world feeling more complete and less frayed around the edges.

Mindfulness with & Because of Others

Mindfulness

FOR WHEN SOMEONE DOESN'T LIKE YOU

It's not in your head. Well, I don't know you, so maybe it is, but my point is that many people can pick up the symptoms of dislike more easily than they could diagnose a cold.

We don't want to confront our family members or our coworkers, so we show up to the holidays and the board meetings and we try to tell ourselves that their thin smiles and eye rolling are directed to everyone. It's not just us.

Or is it?

It is one thing to work on the concept of loving-kindness when someone is easy to love. It is quite another when someone doesn't get us, or even worse, does get us and chooses to dislike us anyway.

Maya Angelou is often quoted as saying, "Forgive everybody," but she also said, "When someone shows you who they are, believe them the first time." The line between these two is the one I try to straddle. To forgive the people who don't like me without having to invite them to my dinner table. To wish them well, without making sure that I am leading myself to *dukha*, or "bad space" (the pre-Taylor Swift "Bad Blood").

If you feel the remnants of someone's dislike, take a seat. Man, you need it.

Sit and breathe in silence for a while, noticing how many thoughts and emotions run underneath each breath. Take a moment to think of all of the people who are easy to love. Let them into your heart. Feel the quality of your experiences with them.

When you feel ready (and this can take a while), shift your focus to the difficult person in your life, the one who doesn't like you. Do your best to stay away from storytelling; you don't have to recap the relationship. You already know the relationship, but start to feel how your body reacts to this relationship. How do you physically feel when you think of this relationship? Are there parts that tighten, that become rigid? Tune into that.

We are not expecting miracles with meditation, we are expecting progress. For me, when I sit like this, I can sometimes feel the tiniest, smallest part of myself melt. There are still parts of me that refuse to yield and parts of my ego that feel too bruised to work toward healing. But still, a small part softens. That is something. That is love. That is the hardest kind of love.

When you feel that tiny shift, open your eyes. Forgiveness is a great gift. Being good at loving is a skill that you have to refine again and again.

Mindfulness

FOR WHEN YOUR COWORKERS ARE GETTING ON YOUR NERVES

Your coworkers are like family. You don't choose them, but you love them anyway. Until you don't.

There are times when you show up to work and the fact that your officemate is playing "Gangnam Style" five years too late is grating on your nerves. Or the "friend" that you know secretly talks behind your back asks how you are doing and you think, *really*?

If you aren't careful, workplace tension can be fraught with as much tension as Thanksgiving dinner. Use this time to do a super fast *metta* meditation to build compassion. It doesn't take long, and suddenly you will realize how much of your frustration may be coming from an inner space. If meditating at your desk isn't yet kosher, take the time in the bathroom to do it, or as one of my students does, go to your car on your break. It is a contained and easy place that will support your spiritual development.

As you close your eyes, think, *may you be happy*, *may you be well, may you be at peace.* Direct these statements to yourself, slowly within your mind. As with any mantra, repeat it often enough until it feels true and real. You can even start to distill the phrase to its easiest components: Happy. Well. Peace.

Now think about the coworkers you are struggling with and start to direct those same phrases toward them. It may take a little longer, but keep with it. Take a minute or two to sit with their image. There may be a lot of things that stand in their way of exhibiting these qualities, but you aren't going to be one of them. Continue to do this with as many coworkers as you are struggling with. Return to work with a lighter heart and an open-minded attitude. As you become more peaceful, it will become harder and harder for people to get under your skin. However, if they do, this meditation will be waiting for you.

Mindfulness

FOR WHEN EVERYONE AROUND YOU IS STRESSED

Ever come back home feeling amazing, only to find that your partner is down in the dumps? It may feel like you are a balloon that is slowly deflating. Or have you ever arrived at work after a flawless commute only to find that a looming deadline is making all of your coworkers crazy?

At times like these, it can be hard to direct your inward energy outward. If the majority of your connections are stressed, it can be too easy to their feel negative outward energy seeping inward.

Is stress contagious?

Not officially, but it sure can feel that way. Two actions are always going on at one time. There is a contracting energy and an expanding energy. There is a world of action and inaction, of stress and complacency.

Even though at some points in time it may feel easy to assume that *everyone* is stressed and *everything* is imbalanced, it is important to realize that extremes are highly unlikely. It is more likely that we are viewing the world through our foggy lens, and we need to bring out the lens cleaner to see that there is more than one side.

Begin to bring your attention to your breathing, deepening your breath as you go. Feel the presence within you expanding. Take a moment to think of someone who brings you great gratitude. Then think of something that brings you great gratitude. Feel the way the body responds to these thoughts.

Don't worry if stress seeps in. It's all in the balance. Come back to deeply breathing into your belly. Come back to recognizing that there is another side, a lightness of being and a clarity that is available to you. This can take mere moments. You may need to step aside to stand on your own side. Do what you have to do to keep the equilibrium and to come home to your center.

Mindfulness

FOR WHEN YOUR PARTNER IS SNORING

You love your partner. He or she knows how to make you laugh and gives the best, most soul-affirming hugs. If only he or she would just shut up. (At night. I mean at night.)

It can be a tough relationship conundrum when your partner wakes up in the morning bright-eyed and bushy tailed (although the bushy tail part should be checked out by a doctor) and you wake up silently furious that they have destroyed your precious beauty sleep.

"Good morning, darling!" *Is it?*

If you are contemplating separate bedrooms or even a swift kick to your partner's shins, it is time to get meditating. Meditation is not going to stop you from hearing, but it will help you stabilize your reactions. While the snoring may be frustrating, what affects you most is what happens *after* the sounds start. You may start freaking out inside, wondering what you are going to do if your sleep dwindles.

This we can do something about.

When you first hear the drone of your partner, don't fight it. The more you push away the noise, the more it will bother you. It is there. Acknowledge it. Some people have to fight with the noise inside their own minds and you have to grapple with the noise outside of your body.

While you notice the noise, begin to take a deep breath in for a count of four. Hold the breath for a count of seven. Breathe out for a count of eight. Is the snoring distracting you? Don't worry about it. Come back to the breath. Count four in, seven to hold, and eight to exhale. Holding the breath in will help to relax the nervous system. Some people believe that this technique can get an agitated person to sleep in sixty seconds or less. It's worth trying. If not, there is also the life hack known as earplugs.

Mindfulness

FOR WHEN YOUR MOTHER-IN-LAW WON'T LEAVE YOU ALONE

It is a lucky thing to marry into another family. To have a bonus family that you can love and nurture. This may be how you felt on your wedding day.

Then life unravels, and just like your family, your spouse's family proves that they are not so perfect. They have their quirks and their quibbles. They refuse to bend and you have to do contortionist moves to fit in.

And then there is your mother-in-law.

Mothers-in-law can be lovely, but it can be difficult to set boundaries with them in the same way you would with your actual mother. If you are tired and your mother calls, you may not answer the phone. The same situation with the suffix "in law" and you may feel compelled to answer.

The main stress with in-laws is the lack of boundaries. The next time you find yourself getting irked, check in with whether it is the person themself who is bothering you or the fact that you haven't established or communicated your personal needs. Even with relationships that are dripping with obligations, we still have every right to draw a line in the sand.

If you are still awash with frustration, allow yourself to recognize that there is no relationship that is fixed. To relate to other people, we must embrace the continuum.

Take a seat and place your hands over your heart. Take many moments to fall in love with yourself, no matter how silly that may seem. Feel the accumulation of all of your qualities that add up to a spectacular human being. Give back. Delight in your own existence.

When you feel like your cup has been filled, come back into the world. The one with in laws and the art of relating. Try to become acquainted with your mother in law, rather than assuming that you already know her. Allow her to surprise you, but only after you have given to yourself.

Mindfulness

FOR WHEN YOU JUST DUMPED SOMEONE

Even when we know things aren't working, it takes courage to say things out loud. People stay in relationships that have hit an end point of growth from days to years longer than they should. I have heard the phrase, "But maybe it will get better!" from far too many of my friends. Optimistic? Maybe. But there comes a point when optimism clouds reality.

Placing an end to a relationship that at one point felt right can put you at odds with yourself. It can feel yucky. It is hard to hurt someone, and in many cases, splits do not end amicably. There is fighting and tears and residue that makes you feel uncertain if you will ever find love again.

I can't predict when and if romantic love will charge in your direction, but I can give you this meditation to help to settle your weary heart.

Have a seat and close your eyes. Focus on your breathing, rippling from your belly to your chest and back from your chest to your belly. There may be emotions that ride with the deep breaths and that is okay. Keep returning to the simplicity of the breath.

Imagine that the air you are inhaling is emerald green. This is the color of the *anahata chakra*, which is the heart chakra and sometimes translated as "unstruck" or "unhurt." The anahata chakra opens us up to the fact that our grievances and past hurts do not define us. At our spiritual cores, we cannot be broken.

As you sit, try not to intellectualize your experience. It is just you, your breath, and the color green. It is the beating of your green heart. You don't need to judge what you did or didn't do. You just need some time to heal, and it starts here.

Mindfulness

FOR WHEN YOUR SIGNIFICANT OTHER DOESN'T PULL THEIR WEIGHT

When you are young and in love, you never think you will be one of "those couples." You will always appreciate one another and have mind-blowing sex. You will never grumble at your partner's inability to pick up their own socks. It's not a big deal, after all. You will just pick up the socks! Forever! Because you're in love!

Things change.

All of us have something that we prefer done a certain way. You may like to separate the laundry while your significant other (SO) couldn't care less. You may not need to make your bed in the morning while your beloved can't start their day with still-creased sheets. Your SO says that they are going to do the dishes, but the next morning you wake up to find them all piled next to the sink, still dirty—this is a common time to lose your shit.

But not you. You are mindful.

The first thing to be mindful of, in this moment, is that change takes time. Just because your SO doesn't see the world the way you do, doesn't mean that a) they don't want, or b) they won't in the future. The trickiest part of a long-term relationship is assuming that the years together are an indication that you can predict their future behavior. Change is hard and change takes time. But if you are capable of it, so too is your SO.

Before you go all crazypants on your beloved, repeat the following at least ten times. "I am hopeful." Hope and anger can't coexist. Hope allows your mind to broaden and think of the big picture, which is a much more positive landscape than assuming everything will be as it is right now. Once you feel calmer and more hopeful, go up to your SO. "Honey? I think you forgot to do the dishes." At the very least, the outcome will be much more positive than negative.

Mindfulness
WITH YOUR PET

If you have a pet, you may notice that they're interested in your meditation practice. Animals are attracted to tranquil energy and you may hear gentle purring or sighing coming from their corner as you sink into stillness. I have taught many private yoga classes that end with my clients and their pets blissfully lying on the ground. Animals understand energy and they are especially drawn to the shifts in their beloved owners.

The next time you decide to meditate, call your cat or dog to be near you. Place one hand on them as you close your eyes. This physical connection is deeply soothing to your animal and a great stress reliever for you.

Focus on your breath going in and out, as well as the gentle rise and fall of the breath you can feel in your pet's body.

If the volume of your pet changes, or if they move around and try to get your attention, try to keep still and centered. They are a great example that even after connecting with calm, the world may have other plans.

Stay with your animal as long as you can, breathing in and out and radiating your serenity in their direction. When the meditation has finished, open your eyes and give your co-meditator a well-deserved belly rub. You've finally spoken a language that he or she understands.

Mindfulness
FOR SEXY TIMES

Apparently, meditation and sex have a lot in common. Do I have your attention? Thought so.

Studies suggest that the brain acts similarly to meditation as it does to sex. Both dissolve our self-awareness and both light up the right hemisphere of the brain, which is nonverbal and creative. The more you meditate, the more you are connected to this portion of the brain.

This is the kind of science that certainly would interest a high schooler who was zoning out in biology class.

We're often blunting our awareness through work, alcohol, or constant activity. Slowing down and connecting to yourself is an exercise in heightened awareness and sensuality. Your current or future partner will certainly enjoy the fact that you're doing, rather than thinking. There are certainly times that call for that.

Ahem.

To connect to this version of yourself, come to a comfortable seated position. After you close your eyes, take a few breaths in and out through your nose. Feel the way your breath travels through your body, as if it is caressing you from the inside. Feel all of the spaces in the front, back, and sides of your body fill with breath and then slowly release.

Focus on your body. Focus on the feeling of the fabric on your skin. Feel the weight of your clothes. Notice the different temperatures within your body: the heat of your seat connected to the floor, the coolness of your shoulders. Notice which parts of your body feel heavy and which parts feel light. Try not to label your experience or change anything. Do not even change the cadence of your breath.

When you feel your thoughts naturally subsiding and slipping away, congratulations, you are in the right hemisphere! Celebrate by coming back to your breath, opening your eyes, and putting on some sexy tunes.

Mindfulness

FOR WHEN YOUR DOG WON'T POOP

Just to be clear, I don't like to talk about poop. I know that it is important. I know that how often we go matters. I know that it holds even more importance when you are tracking the bowel movements of another being, like, say, your animal or your baby.

I just don't want to hear about it.

Now that I have respectfully gotten that out of the way, let me say that after walking many dogs, I have noticed that as regular as a dog may be, he or she doesn't always go on your schedule. Sometimes it seems like they have a conspiracy, understanding that the longer they put it off, the longer they get to wag their tails outside.

Small fuzzy canine. Strong evolved human. Who is going to win?

Exactly.

You often have better things to do than to intently wait by your dogs behind (and if you don't, please email me so that I can give you the names of many amazing books), but just because you are busy doesn't mean that you have to use this waiting time to cultivate frustration. Having a pet is one of the great joys of life. You can use this time to see the world from their loving eyes. After all, if you can't be nice to your dog, who can you be nice to?

The precursor to meditation is the "coming back." When you are sitting in more formal meditation practices, this often means coming back to your breath. When you are walking your dog, come back to the dog. When you find yourself getting impatient or frustrated, notice your dog's open-hearted tail wagging in front of you. When you find yourself planning your life out, come back to the dog. Ask yourself, "How much can I let go and be in this moment?"

Your dog is a Zen master in a furry package. Likely your dog is one of the easiest loves of your life. Walking your dog can be a mindfulness exercise, and a way to bring you back to what matters.

Even if what matters is taking forever to poop.

Mindfulness

FOR WHEN YOUR KIDS WON'T EAT THEIR VEGETABLES

As we age, we lose our taste buds. You may read that sentence twice, wondering why your kid loves bland food if they are teaming with taste buds. It is because it can be overwhelming to eat. Infants have around 30,000 taste buds spread throughout their mouths. By the time they become adults, only about one-third of them remain.

In other words, your kid is not (only) making a point with their food choices. Eating is an intense experience for them. If you are in the midst of a full-blown war every time you come to dinner, it is definitely time to meditate. You may not be able to control how many pieces of broccoli your kid puts in their mouth. You can, however, determine how calm, cool, and collected you will be before you sit down to the table.

This meditation is for the moments before. I know that your life is likely not a calm Zen temple if you are living with small children, but that doesn't matter. Take some time to nourish your innate self-worth, which will keep you from losing it over a plate of steamed vegetables.

Sit still. Close your eyes. Tell your loved ones you will be a few moments. (This can be done in the bathroom if you really can't get a break.) While you sit, do your best to dissolve your agenda. It is so easy to plan, and as a parent, for much of the day your plans are what make the family tick. Place them to the side and simply notice your inhales and exhales. Your mind may churn with activity. Set a timer for however much time you realistically have. Keep coming back to your breathing, to your inner state, to the degree of serenity that can only come from you taking honest and quiet moments with yourself.

This is not a "by the end of this meditation, your kid will want kale" meditation. It is a meditation that will allow you to practice presence, so that whatever does happen is okay. Or even okay-ish.

Mindfulness

FOR WHEN YOUR KIDS ARE DRIVING YOU CRAZY

You might be a very yogic person who can meditate the sugar out of anyone. But then you have children. If you have buttons, those little bundles of joy sure know how to press them.

If you find your patience going down the potty, take a moment to meditate. You can even do this with small children, although the time may be shorter depending on the kind of day you're having.

Start out by lowering your expectations and be okay with whatever happens. Whether you get thirty seconds or five minutes, relish this alone time. As you sit, address your well-being. Feel your breathing inside your body. Open your inner capacity for observation as you soften your belly.

Be with the breath so that you are defined by it, more than you are defined as your role as parent. Just for now. Observe yourself so that you are more than a reaction. See yourself so that you can create more awareness of your habits and your challenges. Accept yourself as a parent for what you have done. Accept your humanity, which will allow you to be more fully present with your children.

When your children call you back from this focused place, fill yourself with gratitude for your little mirrors. Just as sitting in quiet can make you aware of your light and dark places, so too can your kids. You will get frustrated again. You will become impatient. But you can continue to listen and sweetly accept yourself for the parent that you are in this moment.

Breathe through the overwhelming love. Do it when they nap. Do it when they settle. Connecting to yourself is a great gift that you can give your children.

Mindfulness

FOR NEW PARENTS (WHO AREN'T GETTING ANY SLEEP)

Sleep is the building block of nice people, but when you are a new parent, sleep quickly becomes a rare and precious commodity. Things that used to be a part of your life on a regular basis now seem like leisurely pursuits. None of us are our best selves when we are dragging.

When you don't have time to shower, let alone sleep, meditation may be the last thing on your mind. However, meditation has many benefits, and one benefit is the ability to cope with change. Parenthood may be the most demanding yet rewarding change of all.

If you fell asleep more than once reading those last paragraphs, this meditation is for you. I do appreciate that you may not have much time. The next time your little one falls asleep, whether they are asleep in your arms or in a bassinet, take a deep breath. Take another one. Keep deepening your breath until you feel a little calmer. Look at your infant's expanding belly as she or he sleeps deeply. Mimic this breathing by breathing deeply into the pit of your belly.

Now start to say the words "Sat Chit Ananda" to yourself. *Sat* means "being" in Sanskrit, which can be hard to do when you are given a new life with new responsibility. Try to cultivate being. *Chit* means consciousness. Although you are most likely vigilant with your baby, it can be hard to remain conscious of your own needs. *Ananda* means bliss, like the blisses of the smell of your baby's skin, of change, and your continued commitment to your own happiness.

Repeat these words to yourself for as long as you are able to. Come back to them in the moments when you become overwhelmed or haven't had the chance to nurture yourself. Come back to your breath when you need a calming pause. What better time in life to learn the art of being present than now?

Mindfulness

FOR WHEN YOU ARE BLAMING YOUR SIGNIFICANT OTHER

When you're in a long-term relationship, it's inevitable that at some point you will feel taken for granted. You'll also take that person for granted.

Meditation can help you to love better and to react better. Rather than starting sentences with "Why don't you ever . . . " take time to reflect before speaking. This can be seen as an investment for the sake of your future relationship, and to stop the cycle of loaded remarks.

For a few minutes a day, sit down and reflect on what you want from your relationship. It could be security. It could be companionship. It could be laughter. It may change from day to day.

Rather than letting your mind enter the territory of reviewing what it doesn't have, try to keep your mind still.

Imagine that your partner is everything that you want.

Imagine that everything you need from them, you can give to yourself.

Infuse your body with a feeling of loving kindness toward your partner.

Imagine yourself with them right in the beginning when your relationship felt easy and electric. Sit with that feeling in your heart and feel it expand.

This meditation will not fix all relationship woes, but it certainly can help stop the snarkiness that may erode a loving partnership. Every time you need a reminder of why you are together, start by reminding yourself that you can approach the bumps in the road with a calm attitude. If the ultimate goal is lasting love, this will help you get there.

Mindfulness

FOR WHEN YOU WANT TO INTERFERE IN SOMEONE'S LIFE

You know those times. When your friend is talking about her horrible boyfriend. You nod and appear to be listening, but you're thinking *leave him already!* The words are on the tip of your tongue and you think, *what's the harm in telling her?* Or maybe you're speaking to your boss about an idea that you know through experience won't work, yet you have to let them work it out on their own so you stifle your opinion and shut up. Of course, truth is great in many circumstances. However, blurting it out is not optimal in every situation in order to keep your relationships thriving.

If you know you'll be meeting someone who makes you itch to interfere, take a moment before your encounter with this throat-chakra meditation. Sit in a comfortable space. Quietly to yourself, repeat the mantra "Om Janaha." This mantra is related to the throat chakra. The goal is to connect with our throat chakra, our center of clear communication. This chakra also helps us govern when it's appropriate to speak.

If you become bothered by sounds or distracted by thoughts, just bring yourself back to this mental repetition. Set a timer for at least ten minutes. When it goes off, release the mantra and gently open your eyes.

Go forward with your encounter to interfere less and listen more. Speak the truth but also trust that the person will find their truth in their own time.

Mindfulness

FOR WHEN YOU MISS SOMEONE REALLY BADLY

"Missing someone, they say, is self-centered. I self-center you more than ever."

—Sasa Stanisic, *How the Soldier Repairs the Gramophone*

When you really miss someone, Skype just isn't going to cut it. Longing for them can become a physical experience. You can feel the missing in the same way that you might feel a wound.

If you're experiencing a melancholic longing, meditation doesn't ask you to let go of this. In fact, meditation invites you to sit with it, which will help to prevent you from internalizing it.

Offer this meditation to the person that you miss. Locate the emotion of missing in your body. Witness where it resides and start to invite your breath to travel in and out of that area. You can even place your hand on the part of your body that feels the loss the most profoundly.

After some time, become aware of the softening and opening of your chest wall. Envision your breath traveling directly into the heart space, caressing it. Feel every inhalation increase your sense of being in the heart and each exhalation expand and open the heart.

Move your awareness to the back of your heart and the back of your body.

Feel the open space at the back of your heart.

Let the heart space surround and embrace your physical body.

Admitting how you feel can free you of stored emotion rather than ignoring your feelings and having them wash over you again and again.

Finish your meditation by thanking your person. They have granted you the capacity to love and to feel more deeply.

Mindfulness

FOR WHEN YOU CAN'T REMEMBER YOUR COWORKER'S NAME

True story: I closely worked with someone for years. We got along famously; we even started to move from a professional relationship to a friendship. There was only one problem. I could not, for the life of me, remember her name.

I eventually learned it when I heard someone call her by name, loudly. I was so freaking relieved. If, like me, you have a tough time remembering names, or even remembering where your car keys happen to be, meditation can be an excellent tool to help strengthen your memory. Meditation has been proven to thicken the cerebral cortex, which is responsible for concentration, learning, and memory.

I don't know if it's my meditation practice, but I haven't found myself in this conundrum in years. So just the act of meditating is awesome for memory retention. You could choose any meditation you want. Or if you want to double up, you can work on a meditation that is built for improving your memory. As you close your eyes, take a couple of deep breaths to move yourself away from the busyness of the mind. Then begin to think, "Om Hreem Namah." This mantra is thought to help clear the mind of excess and open you to a higher consciousness. In this higher consciousness, you will have more capacity to remember the things that may be deep-seated. Like that darn name.

As with any mantra, you don't have to beat yourself up if you think around it or on top of it. We multitask all day long, including with our thoughts. The more time you have to repeat the mantra, the slower your own inner dialogue can become, but there is no rush and no goal.

Leave your type A at the door and sit for as long as you can.

If, when you open your eyes, you still can't remember the coworker's name, invent an endearing nickname for them. She likes kombucha? Call her that. Sure, it's weird, but it buys you some time.

Mindfulness

FOR WHEN YOU AREN'T GETTING LAID

Even people who don't believe in chakras know sensations that aren't purely physical. There are sensations in the body related to heartache, and knowing when you have stepped into a dangerous situation. There is also that concrete sensation that happens when you haven't gotten laid for quite some time.

We know the word "hangry," a term to describe someone who is easily angered when hungry. The word "horny" has some similar connotations. If unharnessed, you may find yourself at the whim of any attractive person. You may also find yourself easily irked and more willing to roll your eyes.

Before you head off to hump a tree, it is time to balance your sacral chakra (No, I am not flirting with you.). This second energy center is thought to be located below the navel and above the pubic bone. It is where all of your powerful reproductive organs are. It is not only the center for sexuality but also for relationships and creativity.

This is a center that gives us permission to feel. It is also one of the first chakras, meaning it is related to our base instincts. Any type of seat is a good place to work on this area of your body. Close your eyes and settle in. Begin to direct your breath just below the navel and try to picture the color orange. Breathe in orange and breathe out orange. After a few moments, allow images to appear behind the windows of the eyes. Note them.

Be playful with this meditation. Don't make it into a serious exercise. Allow the creativity of your mind to build on what you pay attention to, what you see, and how you think. Give yourself time. You might need another kind of release after this meditation (ahem) but at the very least this will get your creative, er, juices flowing.

Mindfulness

FOR WHEN YOU DON'T WANT TO FIGHT

There are times when a fight hangs thickly in the air, like cigar smoke. It changes the air in a room, quietly clinging to the walls until something innocuous is said and all bets are off.

Obviously, it's worth communicating when something is profoundly bothering you. However, when a bad day turns into a fight that makes a botched cleaning project seem like a valid end of your relationship, it may be time to take a step back and reevaluate. My partner would be happy to tell you that I used to be horrible at this. I am a fixer. Walking away felt like defeat. He helped me to realize that the pause could be a chance to reevaluate my own reaction.

In this back step, take out your meditation skills to make sure you're not misplacing your annoyance. Sitting down, especially after an emotionally tinged moment, may be a loud thing to do indeed. You may hear "That stupid guy," or "I can't believe she did that," or just be consumed by rage. Don't worry. You won't be here for long.

When you're on high alert, often the most annoying thing someone can do is tell you to relax. This is because the very act of relaxing is quite a big step away from where you are right now. Rather than manufacturing a new emotional state, try instead to breathe. Just breathe.

Breathe in, breathe out, and quiet the frustrated voice in your head. The more charged you are, the longer this will take, but you can do it. It's just a matter of time before you breathe a bad experience right out of your body and mind. It's important that you believe that.

Doing such a meditation will help you keep an experience within itself, rather than letting it bleed into others and make a bad moment a bad day (or week . . . or year). Breathe in, breathe out. Sometimes that's all you have to do.

Mindfulness

FOR GOING TO THE DENTIST

No offense to dentists, but their offices are usually one of the last places people want to be. Meditation may not be able to make the experience a pleasant one, but it can certainly help eradicate the clenching that may result from a visit to the dentist—even before you sit in the chair.

One of the principles of meditation is to feel sensation, but not to cling to any sensation. Everything can arise, even the sensation of someone prodding in your mouth. That will pass.

When you find yourself with a bib around your neck, mouth ajar, think about surrendering. You're already in a vulnerable position—do not create an internal fight.

Then notice yourself. Are you fidgeting or tapping your fingers? Are you gripping your muscles and breathing too quickly? Try to monitor your responses.

You may go in and out of a tense bodily state. Keep checking in. You may be anticipating pain more than you're feeling it.

When you do feel it, try to accept that it is a moment. Feel vibrations, heat, thoughts, and feelings.

Then let it all go.

When you have rinsed your mouth and you're ready to leave, reward yourself with a deep, cleansing breath and let the corners of your mouth turn up.

Mindful Moments of Sleep & Energy

Mindfulness

FOR WHEN YOU JUST CAN'T GET ANY PEACE AND QUIET

There is a reason why yoga studios feel so comforting, and not only because of the shiny happy people that inhabit them (spoken by a perceived shiny happy person). Many of these spaces understand that silence is sacred. There is no religious training requirement to experience the depth that comes with saying nothing at all.

However, going to the studio can be a commitment. There is the getting there and the getting back tacked onto an hour-plus–long class. If we want to find inner peace, we may need to look at places that are a little more convenient in order to make meditation a habit.

I don't know about you, but my home life is not silent. I have a neighbor upstairs who always sounds like she is wearing tap shoes. My cats love to meow and purr as soon as I set out my meditation cushion. Even my considerate partner sometimes yells, "Want to go out tonight?" just as I set my meditation timer.

Although we put "peace" together with "quiet" they are not necessarily pairs. Peace is even in the noise and the everyday. If we can find it there, when we find silence it will be icing on the cake.

The next time you are in the midst of a life that won't shut up, take a moment to close your eyes and start to connect to your surroundings. Connect to everything that is going on. All the sounds of life and the hums of your world.

Try to participate in the exercise of not labeling sounds as "good" or "bad." Step out of your bias of likes and dislikes. There is an underlying silence underneath the noise. Seek it out. Sounds will come and go. There is no need to control sound, and there is also no help in getting stressed about it.

Even when silence is escaping you, notice how your body feels at every moment, from an interruption to the pauses in between distractions. In every moment there is a unique tone that only your ears can pick up.

You can have a sound without a reaction. Notice your breathing and the gentle lift that the inhale provides. Notice the exhale as a coming down and a grounding. Find the underlying stillness in your breath and in your emotions. Among all of the action there is space. Be tender. Refuse to be frustrated with yourself if you get drawn into the disruptions.

We have been trained to follow sound and activity. This is a new training. It is subtle. It is yin-like. It may even be peace-full.

Mindfulness

FOR WHEN YOU WAKE UP IN THE MIDDLE OF THE NIGHT

I am a pretty awesome sleeper. There was a time when I couldn't viscerally understand the concept of insomnia. Why didn't people just stay in bed until they fell back asleep?

However, I am human, and in times of high anxiety, I have woken up in the middle of the night. I remember doing this when I was in University during exam time, thinking, *Oh no, what if I don't get enough sleep? What if I fail the exam? What if no one will hire me because I haven't passed Classic American Literature?* I always passed—and I was always sleep deprived. Thank goodness that as I have gotten older I have acquired some coping mechanisms.

The day version of ourselves might be calm, but there is a quiet anxiety that can lurk at night. We can distract that voice all day long with media and conversations and noise, but night is when the truth comes out. There are many people who claim that they have no back pain during the day but agony wakes them up just as they relax. This isn't surprising. We can overtax our adrenals all day, and when our nervous systems finally get a break, they need a moment to digest our experience. We need to feel our days, both physically and emotionally, and some of us are only giving ourselves the bedtime hours for this.

A preventative measure for waking up in the middle of the night is downtime during the day. Time when you are truly doing nothing. Even if you aren't a meditator (which will certainly change once you finish this book, right?) give yourself five minutes to sit and feel. If the self is always doing and thinking or planning, it will have no training to shut off. Sleep will seem foreign to your body and it will rebel against it.

If you still wake up in the middle of the night and find your "doing" self dramatically planning the rest of your life, tell yourself *not now*. This can become a mantra. Inhale on *not* and exhale on *now*. If your heart is particularly racing, take a deep breath and hold it in for as long as is comfortable (keep in mind that this is not a competition). Exhale long, slow, and deep and hold the breath again as long as you can. If your mind is overactive, it will be hard to get through one of these breaths without interjections of all of the things that you could be doing. Keep trying. Keep at it. Believe that you will be able to get back to sleep.

Because guess what? You can.

Mindfulness

FOR WHEN YOU GET WOKEN UP EARLY

People who come to my yoga classes think that I am the epitome of calm. In that studio and at that time, that may be true. However, there is an exception. There is one situation where I almost never keep my cool, and that is when someone wakes me up.

I do not enjoy this. I have never enjoyed this. My natural bear-like state wants nine hours of sleep and when I am awoken before this (which is true on many days), I am anything but the sweet yoga teacher you all know and love. I am grouchy. When you start your day off with a grouchy mood, you are much more likely to end with a grouchy mood. I can't shift my initial reactions. I can become inquisitive and see what I can do about them through meditation.

If I have started the day with a case of the swears, I then sit down and take five minutes for the inner smile meditation. This Daoist meditation technique is amazingly effective at shifting a sourpuss mood.

Take a moment, seated or lying down, and breathe deeply. Then move your fingers to the corners of your mouth. Lift the corners of your mouth ever so slightly. Release the fingers and try to keep that half smile, without your fingers. Feel how that very slight variation can begin to shift your inner state.

After a few moments, take that same inner smile to the center of your heart. Imagine the same lift, the same half smile happening within. Breathe deeply. Finally, take the same half smile and bring it to the center of your brain. Feel your mind itself smile. Imagine the corners of your mind turning upward. Don't rush yourself. Even just five minutes of this meditation can make me into a more tolerable morning person. Perhaps it can do the same for you.

Mindfulness

FOR A PICK-ME-UP

Perhaps you didn't get much sleep last night. Or for many, many nights. There's a reason the book *Get the F#$k to Sleep* became a *New York Times* bestseller.

Coffee—and concealer—are good, quick fixes for mornings when your shut-eye has been less than optimal. I get that. But meditation may be able to last longer. Just forty-five minutes of meditation can be equivalent to three full hours of sleep.

However, you probably don't have forty-five minutes. And if you do, it will most likely be spent in bed, satisfyingly hitting the snooze button again and again. But even with five minutes of mediation, you can rid yourself of the frustration that can accompany exhaustion.

For this meditation, sit rather than lie down—you know why—in a seated cross-legged position or in a chair. Just don't tempt yourself with a supine position in an exhausted state.

Close your eyes and pay attention to your weariness. Notice if you can feel it in your tissues; in your bones. Is there a particular area that feels more tired than another? If so, focus on this spot.

Imagine a light. Imagine that each time you breathe in you gather this light and send it to this weary area. This light is energizing. It is uplifting. When the area feels bathed in light, move on. Address another area. Keep going until your time is up or until you feel a boost. Move forward with your day—and make sure to hit the hay earlier tonight.

Mindfulness

FOR WHEN YOUR ENERGY IS FADING FAST

Ever have one of those days when your regular energy boosting tricks aren't cutting it? When you feel like having a nap, but your life isn't conducive to being a person of leisure?

Of course you have. You are a human being.

When you are lagging, you may be afraid to meditate. Just sitting up straight may feel like *way* too much work. This is when you must give yourself permission to give in to it. Even if you just have five minutes, giving in to the exhaustion will be much more restorative than fighting it all day.

Once you get an opportunity, make yourself as comfortable as possible. If you can, lie down on a bolster or throw your legs up a wall. Set a timer and just breathe. Let yourself feel depleted. There is such a relief in being honest with how you feel at any given moment. A few moments can help you find quiet and space.

Observe the spreading of the chest as you inhale, then the ribs, then the abdomen. Release tension as you find it with gigantic exhalations. Imagine smoothing out the breath. Let your body be passive.

If you have time to stay longer, by all means, give yourself that time. If your timer has gone off and continuing your day is a pressing matter, then thank yourself for respecting your own boundaries and giving your body a chance to breathe when it needed it most.

Mindfulness
FOR HIBERNATION

If you're staying in tune with the seasons, it's only natural that you feel like hunkering down in the cold months. Even the word hunker implies a nip in the air. Have you ever hunkered in the summer?

I digress.

While you're hibernating, you can use this particular time of year to look within in a more committed way. I like the practice of Jin Shin Jyutsu finger mudras.

The Japanese word *jin* means "human." *Shin* means "heart." *Jyutsu* means "art." Taking into account that energy can flow through the body like blood, we use our fingers as pathways to our consciousness.

Start this meditation by holding onto your right thumb with your left hand.

Take three breaths. Then take your left thumb with your right hand.

Your thumb represents worry. Let any worry come up to the surface.

Do the same exercise with your index finger, which represents fear. Your middle finger represents anger. Your ring ringer represents sadness. Finally, your pinky finger is connected to desires and dreams.

If you find that on a particular day, your mind is very focused on one area of thought/one finger, you can spend your whole meditation on that one finger. Tune in deeply to your impulses and you can feel a freedom that comes from allowing yourself to be just as you are.

You might be amazed at how much clarity and calm arises from holding just one finger.

Mindfulness

FOR WHEN YOU WAKE UP EXHAUSTED

I write this after staying up far too late, even though I knew I was getting up early. Hello, I am a thirty-something who can't always figure out her bedtime.

If you have grossly underestimated the necessity of sleep, this meditation is for you. If unattended, the first day without much sleep can be a manic time. It is important to take a seat and take a breath before you get all Tasmanian devil on the world.

Make yourself comfortable (but perhaps not too comfortable). Close your eyes. Do all the things you normally do when you meditate: focus on your inner state, your breathing, and your body. After a few moments, try to only focus on your skull. Feel the cavities for your eyes and your nostrils. Take a moment to imagine your brain floating within this skull, relaxed in its cerebrospinal fluid.

While you imagine the physicality of your brain, picture it relaxing in the same way a muscle might relax. Sleep is the healing tool for our brain, but you are imagining that your brain is receiving healing energy. While you get distracted (and you will, especially if you are tired), keep coming back to the image of your brain, floating and soft, relaxed and open.

When you feel your heart rate has gone down and your mind has become quieter, you may open your eyes. I'm not saying that you won't still need a cup of coffee, but trust me, this meditation is a good start.

Mindfulness

FOR WHEN YOU JUST CAN'T GET BACK TO SLEEP

A sound woke you up, or you got up to pee, or a persistent thought wouldn't let you rest. Now you're up and your mind is racing. You start thinking thoughts like, *I'm already up. I might as well start my day.*

Except that it's 2 a.m.

The world of adulthood is more awesome than I thought it was going to be when I was little. (I was horrified that adults repeated the word "responsibility" and vowed that I would never stop reading kids' books. Vow kept.) However, the hardest part about being an adult is that we love more. (Let me explain.) Our capacity to love grows as we age, and our capacity to think outside of ourselves grows. If we spent all night in our self-centered thoughts, it would be easier to get back to sleep in our own world, but when our world expands, so too do our potential thought bubbles.

The next time you find yourself awake with no foreseeable escape, allow yourself to exhale through your mouth, imagining that the giant exhalation is relaxing your body even more fully onto your mattress. You're going to have to do this more than once. (Trust me.)

Allow your exhalations to become softer, still imagining that you are relaxing on top of your mattress. As you continue to imagine this, multitask by also imagining your thoughts in balloons. These balloons have strings that you are holding onto. Every time you have a thought, visualize it getting full and moving up above your heavy body, away from you. As you get more and more relaxed, imagine yourself grabbing a giant pair of scissors and cutting the strings of the balloons. Watch the balloons float away from you. Feel the relief of no longer needing to hang on for dear life to your next worry, thought, or idea. Hopefully this will work to send you straight back into dreamland.

Mindfulness in Times of Travel

Mindfulness

FOR PUBLIC TRANSPORTATION DELAYS

I have lived in a lot of different cities all over the world in places that have different languages and different customs. Yet no matter where you are on the planet, there is a universal truth: transportation delays don't bring out the best in people. Even when we see a delay coming, we like to believe that our buses and trains won't fail us. Even a couple of minutes can cause extreme inconvenience, and let's be honest, people who are inconvenienced are not necessarily the best versions of themselves. I can speak with experience after having had to cancel a yoga class because I couldn't make it there on time.

The next time there is a hint of a transportation delay, get proactive. Assume that it will happen. Will you carpool? Can you walk part of the way by getting an early Uber and putting the destination slightly short of where you need to be? For at least part of the time, connect to the sensation of walking. This is a magnificent way to develop focus, bring you into the present, and increase your daily exercise. Try not to change the way you walk at the beginning. Rather than self-correcting, just notice your habits. Where does your foot strike on the ground? How much pressure transfers from one foot to the next?

Try to become aware of the sensations in your feet, from the pressure, to the feeling in your toes, to the feeling of the fabric of your socks. Begin to slowly climb your way up your body, spending at least ten steps with each part: ankles, calves, thighs, and so on until you reach the top of your head. Stay with yourself, even though the world may be speeding past you. When you arrive, take ten seconds to stand in place, feeling the multifaceted balancing act that keeps you upright. Feel the grounding effect in your mind, as well as your body. Thank the universe for the delay that allowed you to stop going through the motions and start feeling what it is like to be you.

Mindfulness

FOR THE POST-VACATION BLUES

If you have taken a true vacation, it may surprise you how much you forget your everyday life. Returning home, the stress may seem palpable. Overwhelming emails, dinners that need to be cooked, and responsibilities around every corner.

Where the hell are the palm trees and the gentle breezes? Is this really your life?

You don't want to undo the benefits of time off right away. Having lived in vacation destinations, let me tell you, the magic wears off after a while. Vacations simply feel magical because they are unique.

However, that doesn't mean you can't bring some of that vacation home.

I am not suggesting you pick up more souvenirs. Nix the magnets and instead bring something that evokes a very simple memory through one of your senses. It could be the hotel soap. It could be the feeling of sand. It could be the song that kept playing when you woke up from an outdoor nap.

Once you are home and feel any post-vacation longing, take a moment with your object. Use the sense that you most associate with this object. Try not to drown in nostalgia. Simply be with the emotions and the physical state that this fragment of your vacation carries with it.

Although this may seem like an exercise in sitting in the past, if you take enough time, you will catapult yourself into the present. You will notice the simple pleasures of the everyday and the beauty that is around you. Transcend the object and sit for a few minutes, without relaying your do-to list or even your vacation memories. Just sit, knowing that you can be productive later. Right now, the most productive thing you can do is enjoy being alive.

Mindfulness

FOR TURBULENCE

I have several techniques to help me through airline turbulence, because I don't like it. I travel a lot and I used to travel excessively. Even so, I never got to the point of enjoying a bumpy ride. I recognized that although white-knuckling the seat is one solution, it's not the only one.

It's good to know that the airplane wants to return to its positive stability. Turbulence is not a premonition of a crash, but rather a nuisance that may spill your coffee. Even so, you may feel precarious and fragile at 35,000 feet in the air. I totally get it. So let's get prepared in advance.

Prior to your flight, purchase a bar of chocolate. Not that cheap stuff you can get in the airport, but something sumptuous and expensive and delightful. The kind of chocolate you rarely treat yourself to because it's just too much. Pack that treat in your carry-on. It is not there to pass the time at the airport. It is your emergency chocolate meditation.

Once you are at altitude, lie back and enjoy the ride. If things get bumpy, take out your chocolate. Take a piece and smell it. Place that piece in your mouth and enjoy the sensation. Notice the different layers of flavor, both subtle and obvious. Hold the chocolate in your mouth for as long as possible and allow it to melt. While you are eating your chocolate, think the mantra, *I choose calm*. This has helped me immensely. You may not be able to choose the air currents, or whether or not your flight is late, but you certainly can choose calm.

Once the piece is over, see if the turbulence has subsided. If not, take out another piece and linger with your senses and repeat to yourself, *I choose calm*. This may be one of the most enjoyable forms of mindfulness meditation out there. Because chocolate.

Sure, turbulence may not be your favorite experience. But a few pieces of chocolate on their own can calm the nerves, and when you use them to meditate, you'll come off the plane with reduced levels of stress hormones. You have arrived.

Mindfulness
FOR JET LAG

When you're crossing time zones, you may start to notice that things get a little fuzzy. Whether you're feeling dizzy or just plain exhausted, the lack of synchronization between your inner and outer world can bring you into a strange headspace.

The best way to deal with jet lag is to not get it. Put yourself on the time of your destination as soon as you are on the flight. When it hits the time that you should be sleeping, start to close your eyes. Think to yourself, *I am free of jet lag*. The mind is a very powerful thing. Our experiences are an outer manifestation of our thoughts and beliefs, and what we plug into can determine how we react.

You can say this many times in your head, even if you start out not believing it. It can help to reprogram your attitude. Be mindful of your body, even if it is smushed into an airplane chair. Breathe in and out. Try not to predict what your trip will be like or review the work that you still need to do.

Find one part of your body that is relaxed (it could be your nose). Focus your energy on this area for as long as possible, returning to it when you get distracted. As you tune in, try to imagine spreading this relaxation to different parts of your body. Don't rush yourself and expect that this can be done within minutes. If you have a long flight, you also have a long time to meditate. Even if you can't sleep, meditation can help to make up for some of the deficiency. Without that pesky jet lag, you can enjoy your new location even sooner. Bon voyage!

Mindfulness
ON THE SUBWAY

I have never owned a car. Now that I am a proper adult, it seems no more likely to happen, which means I will be spending more time on public transportation.

Hurray?

With transportation strikes, delays, and bad weather, it is not always the most enjoyable way to get around. I know that I am not alone. Many of us commute to get from point A to point B, point B being the place that affords us the subway pass in the first place. During rush hour, you likely would use the word "relaxing" for your commute about as frequently as you would call your fellow passengers "charming." You may not get a seat. You may be stacked against people like bumper-to-bumper traffic (and guess who one of those bumpers is).

How can you meditate here?

First, stop trying to do more. As you get to your destination, stop trying to hold a paper and getting frustrated when the subway lurches. Just stand. Or sit. This is the essence of meditation.

Try to prevent your frustrations from overcoming you, or from letting your eyes aimlessly drift along the posters. Keep your eyes fixed with a soft gaze (preferably not on a person, because that's just creepy).

Keep your feet firmly planted. Ride the waves of the subway, engaging your core like you're on a surfboard. Every time you get to another stop, remind yourself: Breathe in. Breathe out, and take a really good, deep breath from the bottom of your belly, and repeat. Soft gaze, ride the wave, breathe in, breathe out. If you want an additional challenge, you can record the number of seconds an inhale takes, and increase it as you get to each stop.

When you reach your stop, start walking to your destination. Be confident in the fact that you have the tools to keep calm and carry on.

Mindfulness

FOR WHEN YOU CAN'T FIND A PARKING SPOT

Around and around she goes . . .

I am not a regular driver, which means that when I drive, I expect everything to go perfectly. (And we all know how things go on the road—and in life—when expectations are sky-high.) Parking doesn't bring out the best in people. It is the adult equivalent of a toddler screaming "*Mine*!" We avoid eye contact. We cut people off. We panic on our fifth circle around the lot. What a great opportunity to be mindful.

While you are in the car moving at this slow pace, begin to imagine warm embers stoking a fire in the center of your heart. Lest you associate the fire with anger, allow the fire to be soft and glowing. This fire represents your kindness toward yourself and toward the world around you.

Parking is the ultimate practice of what yogis call "aparigraha," which means non-grasping. Can you search for what you need without becoming jealous of what someone else has found? (This is why yoga is seen as a practice—it isn't easy!) As you continue to circle the parking lot, allow that warm, kind feeling to flow through your entire body. Rather than becoming tense and frustrated due to the repetitive nature of the task, let parking be an opportunity to pause and connect you with the parts of you that are patient and kind and soft, no matter how people are reacting around you.

It is so easy to get pulled into mass emotion. It is a work in progress to stand alone and to be firm in your core values. If you work on this mindful mini, once you do find your parking space, you will be able to exit your car feeling grounded and relaxed. Frazzled is *so* not who you are.

Mindfulness

FOR WHEN SOMEONE CUTS YOU OFF ON THE ROAD

Driving tends to either be very good or very bad. Either you are channeling your inner Jerry McGuire by singing *Free Falling* as the breeze flows through your gorgeous hair or someone is giving you the finger right after you swerved and spilled your coffee on your white shirt.

Of course, there is the middle ground, getting from point A to point B. Intrinsically, we know we can't control the people in our lives, let alone strangers. Yet put any of us behind a wheel and we become aggravated by smart cars and gas guzzlers alike.

Why don't they watch where they are going?

There is enough vitriol in the world, and when you find your blood boiling by someone's driving, you are the only one left with that feeling. That person may momentarily feel embarrassed, or they may not even notice. If you drive often and find your blood pressure rising at the fact that you can't control other people, it is only hurting you.

Here is a mindfulness exercise I have done when someone has sped past me, or cut me off unexpectedly. Rather than assuming the worst about that person, I do quite the opposite. I assume the best. That person may have just been fired from their job, or rushing to the hospital to their dying mother, or distracted because they had just heard the words, "I don't love you anymore."

This life thing is tough, and it can be tough on all of us.

After the person has zoomed away without noticing me, I choose to notice them. I do a simple loving kindness exercise. "May you be happy. May you be well. May you find peace." I then take a deep breath and as I exhale, I imagine this exhale helping to relax this person and make them believe that they will be okay.

I am well aware that some people may be entitled or self-centered or unaware. However, contributing to a life of compassion feels far more empowering to me than allowing my inner ogre to win.

Mindfulness

FOR RUSH HOUR TRAFFIC

No matter how Zen of a person you are, rush hour traffic can beat you down. The honking of cars with slack-jawed people behind the wheels can make the extension of a commute seem like the least meditative part of any day.

The next time you are crawling by at a snail's pace in traffic, try to do an open-eyed meditation.

(Please. Keep your eyes open.)

Turn off the drone of the radio and let the reduced noise help you. The city still may sound like an out-of-tune symphony around you, but in your car, the world is quieter.

Now notice if your emotions toward the rush hour traffic are having any physical effect on your body. You may notice that your breathing is jagged, so take a few deep breaths, even letting that breath come out of your mouth. (Hey, it's no weirder than that nose picker in the car beside you.)

Notice if there is anger or frustration presenting itself within the belly or as a tight band around the chest. Look within as you continue to look out. Have the external environment around you be external, trying to be conscious to not absorb any of it into your internal environment.

The longer you're stuck bumper to bumper, the more opportunity you have to practice self-reflection and arrive at your destination, cool as a cucumber.

GLOSSARY OF TERMS

APARIGRAHA

Aparigraha is part of one of the eight limbs of yoga, the *yamas*, which relates to how we conduct ourselves in our day-to-day lives. Aparigraha specifically relates to non-grasping, which is a pretty important concept in our current world. Working on non-grasping assures that we are not spending all our waking hours in fervent desire of the new iPhone.

CHAKRA

When I first learned about chakras, I rolled my eyes more than I listened. Spinning vortexes of energy did not resonate with me on any level, but I figured I would have to suffer through the lectures in order to become a yoga teacher. However, as I delved more into Eastern philosophy, it made sense to me on my own terms.

Here is how I see it: we have the part of our bodies that is anatomical, and the part of our bodies that is emotional. When you experience emotional heartbreak, your actual heart isn't broken, but it can still feel physical. When you get nervous before a presentation, you don't actually have butterflies in your stomach, but it feels real. All of these experiences can be explained within the chakra system. It is as if there is a particular charge and energy that can be balanced or out of whack within each part of our body. We can store our emotional experiences the way we can store tension in our backs.

Of course, we are all incredibly different. Some of us relate more to sounds than concepts. Others to colors. Chakras have a lot of different jumping off points and just like meditation, they won't all work for you, but one area might. Here are the seven chakras and some of the key information that relates to them.

ROOT CHAKRA (BASE OF THE SPINE)

- Related to feeling at home in different situations and within yourself.
- Sanskrit name: *Muladhara*
- Color: red
- Sound: lam

SACRAL CHAKRA

- Related to emotions, creativity, and passions.
- Sanskrit name: *Svadhisthana*
- Color: orange
- Sound: vam

NAVEL CHAKRA

- Related to self-esteem, power, and assertiveness.
- Sanskrit name: *Manipura*
- Color: yellow
- Sound: ram

HEART CHAKRA

- Related to love (including self-love), courage, compassion, and connection.
- Sanskrit name: *Anahata*
- Color: green
- Sound: yam

THROAT CHAKRA

- Related to how your truth relates to your speech and your power of expression.
- Sanskrit name: *Vishudha*
- Color: blue
- Sound: ham

THIRD EYE CHAKRA (IN BETWEEN THE EYEBROWS)

- Related to intuition, insight, and imagination.
- Sanskrit name: *Ajna*
- Color: indigo
- Sound: om

CROWN CHAKRA

- Related to your feeling of connectivity with the rest of the world as well as your spiritual beliefs.
- Sanskrit name: *Sahasrara*
- Color: purple
- Sound: om (Already makes those "oms" in yoga seem a little more powerful, doesn't it?)

DUKHA

The first of the Four Noble Truths in Buddhism and found in the Upanishads in Hinduism, *dukha* translates roughly to "bad space" or "suffering."

EIGHT LIMBS

In Patanjali's Yoga Sutras, the eight limbs are the steps to a meaningful life driven by yoga (and not the Lululemon-clad version we know today). These include our own integrity through nonviolence, truthfulness, non-stealing, the right use of energy, and non-grasping.

It also includes self-discipline such as cleanliness, contentment, spiritual commitment, study of the self, and the ability to surrender to something greater than ourselves. Finally, it delves into the yoga postures, yoga breathing, and other techniques to become free (withdrawal of the senses, concentration, meditation, and a state of oneness).

INNER SMILE

A self-healing and nurturing Taoist meditation practice.

ISHA KRIYA

In Sanskrit, a *kriya* is an internal action, and *isha* is the source of creation. *Isha Kriya* is a meditation technique which was developed by the yogi and mystic Sadhguru as a way to enhance clarity and reduce stress.

JIN SHIN JYUTSU

A Japanese healing philosophy that works as a form of acupressure to unlock twenty-six energy points in the body. It roughly translates to "The art of the creator through compassionate man."

MANTRA

A word or sound repeated to help with concentration in meditation. It is often used in Hindu and Buddhist traditions.

METTA

This is a loving kindness meditation to help the practitioner direct well-wishes to other people.

PARASYMPATHETIC NERVOUS SYSTEM

One of three divisions of the autonomic nervous system and the one that is often tapped into during a meditative practice. The heart rate slows and blood pressure decreases: a state often referred to as "rest and digest."

SUKHA

The opposite of *dukha*. *Su* is good and *kha* is space in Sanskrit. *Sukha* can be translated to "ease" or "bliss" and is seen as a feeling of deep, lasting contentment.

VIPASSANA

Insight meditation within the Buddhist tradition. Rather than distracting oneself, vipassana focuses on removing the cloaks that prevent us from truly seeing ourselves. It makes us more aware and if we get it down, we become liberated. (I'm still working on that one.)

ACKNOWLEDGMENTS

I am a grateful person, so bear with me.

Firstly, thank you to my esteemed Skyhorse editor Nicole Mele, who believed in this book and guided me patiently through the process of publishing it. You are both kind and efficient, and those things don't often go together.

Thank you to my tuja wellness editor, Kyla Gaertner. You stretched my writing more than I thought was possible and your words of encouragement still sit with me years after we worked together.

To Maureen Johnson, one of my early babysitters and encouragers who took my ideas seriously, edited my early work, and spent hours with me in bookstores before I was tall enough to reach the shelves.

To Mrs. Nazarewycz, the first teacher who saw through my shyness and stood up for me, making me stand up for my poetry even when bullies tried to make me smaller.

For my yoga students who let me into their hearts and allowed me to be taught by them. Getting quiet together has been a gift for me as much as you.

For the dear friends I have made in the last ten years who have brought me tea when I was sad and joined me in my joy. Knowing you constantly stokes my heart. The fact that you live all over the world makes me feel more connected to everything.

To my mom, dad, and sister, who didn't laugh when I declared at age ten that I wanted to write a book, and loved me even when I was at my least lovable.

To my animal loves Alfred and Venus, for keeping my lap warm when my creativity burns low and for showing me that self-improvement is not just for humans.

Finally, to the most important person in my life. Mike, you are my best friend. I can't imagine not waking up next to you, not laughing with you, and not growing with you. Your love makes everything possible, including the remarkable Theodore.